Death, Disease & Dissection

Death, Disease & Dissection

The Life of a Surgeon-Apothecary, 1750–1850

Suzie Grogan

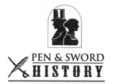

PEN & SWORD
HISTORY

First published in Great Britain in 2017 by
Pen & Sword History
an imprint of
Pen & Sword Books Ltd
47 Church Street
Barnsley
South Yorkshire
S70 2AS

ISBN 978 1 47382 353 2

A CIP catalogue record for this book is
available from the British Library.

Printed and bound in England
by CPI Group (UK) Ltd, Croydon, CR0 4YY

Pen & Sword Books Ltd incorporates the Imprints of Pen & Sword Books
Archaeology, Atlas, Aviation, Battleground, Discovery, Family History, History,
Maritime, Military, Naval, Politics, Railways, Select, Transport, True Crime,
Fiction, Frontline Books, Leo Cooper, Praetorian Press, Seaforth Publishing,
Wharncliffe and White Owl.

For a complete list of Pen & Sword titles please contact
PEN & SWORD BOOKS LIMITED
47 Church Street, Barnsley, South Yorkshire, S70 2AS, England
E-mail: enquiries@pen-and-sword.co.uk

For Peter, always.

Contents

Acknowledgements

Many people have offered support in the writing of this book but I would particularly like to thank the staff at the Wellcome Library and The London Library for their expertise, and the libraries themselves for offering a wonderful space in which to work on my research trips to London.

A special thank you to John Ford MD FRCP who contacted me on behalf of the Society of Apothecaries and pointed me to some little-known but important biographies of interesting men of the period, and to Mike Rendell, not only a 'Georgian Gent', but a gentleman in the true sense of the word who offered his terrific knowledge of the period and lent me some very precious, original documents to photograph for this book.

Once again, I have been away on a number of occasions to concentrate on writing this book, and would like to send my love and thanks to my great friend Cornelia Marock and her family, who invited me to stay with them in Liechtenstein for a week of writing, when it looked as if I would never finish the manuscript. My daughter, Evie, also put me up, or put up with me, on research trips to London, which I know rather cramped her style. Thank you darling.

Thank you to my friends Sarah Whittingham, Angela Buckley and Gill Hoffs who have, at various times (and probably without knowing it) inspired me to keep writing and supported me when the task felt overwhelming. I wish them all very good luck with their own books, to be published in the coming months.

Sincere thanks to all at Pen and Sword for their hard work in bringing this book to publication, and a special mention for my husband Peter, for his endless patience, proofreading skills and constant supply of strong coffee.

Introduction

In the twenty-first century, we talk about going to see 'our GP' as a first point of contact when we have a health worry. How many of us stop to consider, however, that the men and women, we make an appointment to see, are members of a long line of hard-working doctors who have been treating our minor health concerns and signposting us to other services for the more serious conditions, for more than 200 years? That their forbears were eighteenth and nineteenth century surgeon-apothecaries and a mixed band of practitioners, from the powerful physician and surgeon to the horse doctor and local 'nurse', working with what few tools they had to make us well?

The doctors of the late eighteenth and early nineteenth century were regularly lampooned in cartoons of the period as men willing to feed the worst fears of their patients and take their wealthy and 'worried-well' patients for every penny they could squeeze out of them. The patients, too, were often seen as hypochondriacs with more money than sense, willing to try any weird and wonderful, but probably useless, preparation to cure themselves of an imagined ill, or the results of their overindulgence and dissipation.

In this book, I wanted to move away from that frequently bewigged stereotype and highlight some of the hard-working and idealistic men who, often by luck, have had their story noted down somewhere, and their diaries and ledgers uncovered for the wonderful social history they contain. At the same time, I wanted to address the context, the medical world within which they worked and the difficulties they faced. There were many practical obstacles, from affording apprenticeships and further training, to the social prejudice many of them faced throughout their working lives. From the late eighteenth-century Poor Law regulations, which allowed some of them to build up a practice that paid, to the post-1834 new Poor Law changes, which took away much-needed income and made it harder for the dedicated doctor to treat the poorest in his parish? What competition did they face? What conditions could they treat, and with what? What changes did they see in that period of great industrial upheaval and enlightenment thinking?

Chapter 1 looks at the structure of medicine in the period covered by this book – 1750 to 1850 – and notes how the different 'class' of medical practitioner was social as well as professional. The university trained doctor or 'physician' of the day may, in fact, know far less practical medicine than his surgeon or apothecary counterparts, but they were more likely to be invited into fashionable society. (An exception perhaps is surgeon-apothecary Henry Jephson, in Chapter 7.) The social niceties of medicine are fascinating and the arguments between, and within, the different colleges could go to extremes.

At what point did the surgeon-apothecary appear, and when had he fully metamorphosed into the general practitioner? Irvine Louden in *Medical Care and the General Practitioner* offers an academic perspective on the period, with a vast array of statistics and detailed examination of the medical changes, and has found the first reference to 'general practitioner' in a letter by one 'H' written in 1809. He feels it isn't important to be specific about the dates but that, in this more general history, the change was almost complete by the end of the period and seems to be a label that changed as society changed; from the remnants of the mystical medicine of rural lives long past, to the mechanised, practical society of the industrial revolution and the reign of Queen Victoria. Medicine progressed in giant leaps as anaesthesia was identified, as the true causes of epidemics and the transmission of infection were recognised, and as doctors discovered there were ways that medicine, as well as surgery, could cure rather than just control. The label described the man, and eventually, it would describe the woman too.

Medical treatment and cure, rather than palliative medicines, were in their earliest stages of development in this period. There were no antibiotics of course, and no anaesthesia until towards the middle of the nineteenth century. The surgeon-apothecary would have been faced with many patients suffering a fever without any hope of identifying the cause so, despite the doctor's best efforts, his treatment was often ineffective. He was there to offer comfort and reassurance, to give confidence to the patient and family, in the hope that it may aid recovery.

Conditions behind a general sickness were mainly unidentified – diabetes, for example, was not identified until 1889, and it can cause a variety of symptoms that are easy to treat today but would have mystified many 200 years ago. Heart conditions could be treated by digitalis, the use of which was identified by William Withering in 1785, but in the early nineteenth century, its use was largely confined to treating oedema (swelling as water collects in the tissues). A lack of Vitamin C had been discovered as the cause of scurvy, and malaria responded to cinchona bark, a source of quinine. Pain could be eased with laudanum (a tincture of opium in alcohol, and highly addictive), and there were various 'cures' for venereal disease. Chapter 5 looks more closely at the practical and medical help a medical man could give, and the remedies at his disposal.

Mortality figures from the period are high. Children died from illnesses easily identified and vaccinated against now – measles, mumps, whooping cough, scarlet fever, chickenpox, diphtheria and German measles. Highly infectious smallpox, typhus, malaria and meningitis could kill in large numbers, and puerperal (post-natal) fever was something new mothers feared, and which seemed a fact of life until it was discovered, partly by one of the men featured in this book, to be caused by the doctor's poor practise. Epidemics, such as cholera and typhoid could ravage whole communities, and the cause of many of these lethal conditions would not be understood until the end of the period covered by this book. In 1800, the average life span of an adult in Britain was just 48 years of age.

Theories relating to the balancing of the body's 'humours' (blood, yellow bile, black bile and phlegm), and the miasma or 'bad air' theories of disease transmission were being challenged, but at this point, there was little evidence of any real alternative. So treatments for many medical conditions still involved an attempt to 'rebalance' the body by expelling poisons or toxic substances. Thus the significant involvement of a patient's digestive system – using an emetic to make someone sick or a purgative to loosen the bowels, alongside the treatment favoured by many physicians – bloodletting by venesection, cupping, and the application of leeches. Many believed that these treatments, used regularly, could act to maintain health, and patients asked their doctors to take pints of blood on a regular basis.

Surgical interventions were often more successful than medical attempts, and the surgeon-apothecary would have spent much of his time treating many of the injuries seen in modern day Accident & Emergency departments. In rural and urban communities, broken bones and crush injuries were commonplace, caused by carts and horses, for example. Gunshot wounds were frequent, especially in rural areas, as were burns and scalds. He could set fractures using plaster and splints (but no anaesthetic) and although many referred the worst cases to specialist surgeons; it was possible they would amputate limbs too. Those who amputated limbs had to work quickly to minimise blood loss and shock.

Many would be surprised to know how common it was for the surgeon-apothecary to act as midwife, and eventually, it became part of their training.

Chapter 4 looks at the controversy caused as the man-midwife of the eighteenth and nineteenth centuries gradually usurped the female midwife, a controversy still discussed by gender historians today. A good midwife was very popular and was regularly booked well in advance of any due date. Care was rudimentary, however, with no antenatal care and little chance of survival should a baby be born prematurely. Childbirth was, after all, not seen as an illness, but as a natural event – and for some doctors a regular nuisance.

However, this book details the work done by men who are little known today, but who recognised that childbirth was more dangerous (although not so lethal as fiction might have us imagine) than it needed to be and who worked hard to identify the cause of puerperal fever, for example.

Readers may be familiar with the description given by Fanny Burney of her mastectomy, or Samuel Pepys of the operation to remove 'the stone' in his bladder – a common complaint throughout the eighteenth and nineteenth centuries, a time when pain could only be lessened by means of alcohol or opiates

Pictures of patients being held down on the operating table, whilst surrounded by a crowd of young medical students keen to learn the latest techniques, both shock and fascinate us, but for a local surgeon-apothecary, these operations would be a rare event, albeit a traumatic one.

The everyday life of a surgeon-apothecary general practitioner during the period 1750 to 1850 is not just a tale of the daily grind – almost literally – of making and prescribing pills and potions. The biographies of the men included in this book offer a picture of how a 15-year-old apprentice could get to the point where he was qualified to take on an important role in the community. His training was long and arduous and explained in relation to that undertaken by the university-trained physician and the 'pure' surgeon, many of whom the would-be surgeon-apothecary could have followed around the wards of the biggest teaching hospitals, and heard at their lectures and demonstrations.

This book includes a chapter on some of the most unpleasant aspects of that hospital training. Unashamedly, there are tales of dissection rooms and resurrection men included, as these were of huge importance to the medical training of the time. In fact, an act of parliament – The Anatomy Act 1832 – was passed to ensure a legal supply of cadavers, enough to end the trade in bodies that led men into churchyards at the dead of night to dig up bodies of the recently deceased. It is not all Burke and Hare, newspapers at the time enjoyed printing discussions between the surgeons and worried members of the public who could sense that the Act was one that would disproportionately affect the poor. Some of the quotes included here are ones that would suit some of the arguments about the welfare bills of the twenty-first century.

The hospitals in which most of these men trained were, for the most part, founded within the period covered, and the network of London hospitals grew dramatically in the eighteenth and nineteenth centuries, as more and more voluntary hospitals were founded to treat the poor (the wealthy always preferred to be treated at home). Some became training hospitals of international repute and are still at the forefront of global medical development today. Hospitals like Guy's in London and Addenbrookes in Cambridge were founded by a wealthy benefactor, or more often a group of benefactors, and run as charitable establishments with rules about who could be admitted – and who could be refused entry, therefore being thrown at the mercy of Poor Law establishments and workhouse infirmaries.

Similarly, the effects of the introduction of the new Poor Law in 1834 are discussed in Chapter 4. Again, there are haunting similarities in the rhetoric used then and now – the 'deserving' and 'undeserving' poor, and the different treatment of those 'poor' and those destitute – the latter seen as rather beyond hope or help, and responsible for their own fate.

We can ask 'who were his peers' and look at the surgeons and physicians of the period, but we must also consider some additional competition for the pennies of the poor, as detailed in Chapter 6; all those known as 'irregular practitioners' – the horse doctors, midwives, nurses with no formal training (and many others who had, informally, offered medical care down the centuries), and, of course, the 'quack'. That term has been used to mean slightly different things and was certainly bandied about by anyone wishing to secure his place as a 'regular' doctor, in whatever field. To them, anyone without the formal training and qualifications could be a 'quack' and were therefore not to be trusted.

In reality, the very poorest would always go to someone who could provide a solution to their ills, or those of their family, at the cheapest cost, and the true 'quack' was more likely to be the seller of patent medicines, which they knew to be useless at best, and poisonous at worst. There are some sad cases of deaths at the hands of these potions, but despite frequent attempts in the media to expose some of these medicines, their ingredients and the manufacturer behind them, they remained incredibly popular as over-the-counter self-care. They brought in taxes desperately needed by the government so there was little incentive to legislate. Some are still available today and do have recognisably useful properties. These include, for example, *Vicks Vaporub* and *Andrews Liver Salts*, which goes to show that medicines may be patent, but they needn't be 'quack'. It was not always an easy distinction to make and as it turns out, many of the least useful medicines were promoted by the biggest names in medicine and used in the major teaching hospitals. But many were made by entrepreneurial spirits, rather than those with real medical knowledge, which could lead to disaster as infants suffered overdoses of laudanum, or were treated with little more than sugar water until the case became too far gone for anyone to treat.

One of the key things this book sets out to do is to bring together some men who are little known today, but who, in their time, made a significant contribution to the lives of those around them – patients, family, and community. Their lives may have been, in some ways, 'ordinary', but they came from contrasting backgrounds, and had contrasting luck in their careers. Robert Storrs, Henry Jephson, Charles Turner Thackrah, Thomas Paytherus, Hampton Weekes and his family, Henry Stephens (who moved from surgeon to ink manufacturer of much fame), and James Parkinson (who first described the symptoms of Parkinson's disease) who inadvertently became involved in a plot to kill George III and ended up hunting dinosaurs.

These were not the men lampooned in the press, and one would hope they never connected themselves with the cartoons that still make us giggle today. On the whole, they were hard-working, well-meaning men who did the very best they could for their patients with little recourse to effective treatments.

John Keats is given significant space in this book, because, owing to his later fame as one of the best of English Romantic poets, there has been considerable examination of his life outside poetry, and that includes a lengthy period as an apprentice to a surgeon-apothecary, and further training at Guy's Hospital in London, where he walked the wards, attended lectures, dealt with the horrors of the dissecting room, and was one of the first doctors to be trained under the provisions of the very important Apothecaries Act in 1815. Biographers have examined his family papers, the one surviving medical notebook, his many letters to family and friends and his poetry to build a picture of the life of (albeit not a typical student) a young man working to pass examinations and learn the practical skills necessary. As I was writing this book, it became clear that Keats was a contemporary of one of the other men included and all that prevents him being the perfect case study is that, thankfully for the English language if not for his patients, he gave up medicine to focus on poetry, never giving up on the thought that one day he might return to it, if only to make some much-needed money.

So, to money, what could a surgeon-apothecary or a general practitioner in a rural area hope to earn per annum? What kind of life did he lead to achieve the sums necessary to keep his family? What steps did men take to create a medical 'dynasty', keeping medicine in the family for decades? What charges did a general practitioner make and to whom? And why was the redrafting of the old Poor Law into the new Poor Law of 1834 such a make-or-break issue for many doctors of the time? For those who made it to the top of their profession, what were the rewards? For those who didn't, were there compensations or just disappointment? Some of these questions are answered in Chapter 4, others are identified in the individual biographies of the men focused on in detail in Chapters 7 and 8. I end the period covered in this book at 1850 because that was the year in which the general practitioners of the day, now largely accepted as the family doctor of first resort, attempted to validate their existence by establishing a College of General Practitioners, to achieve the same status as that of physicians and surgeons. The attempt failed, partly because there was still so much that was unclear about the structure of the medical profession as a whole. Real change and real training came later in the century, along with the admission of women into medical training. Women play minor roles in this book, something I am conscious of and disappointed about. It is a story of herbalists denigrated, midwives usurped and nurses ordered about by young doctors keen to show they knew their stuff. In an attempt to redress that somewhat, Appendix 3 looks at women in medicine at the time and their fight for recognition, which only came to fruition later.

Throughout the research for this book, there were moments when comments made 200 years ago resonated strongly with our present day medical system. General practitioners today have less and less time to spend with individual patients, their lists grow ever longer, and the profession is overstretched and understaffed. Although the early nineteenth-century medical market was technically over-crowded, with a seemingly endless supply of doctors, there was, in fact, fierce competition, a move towards tendering for good positions as they became available and a drive towards squeezing ever more out of a doctor for the smallest possible fee. If one complained, there were many more to take his place.

Arguments about who was responsible for treating which particular class of patient meant some fell through that dreaded 'loophole', as subjective decisions made by more-or-less caring Poor Law Guardians meant the line between the deserving poor and the undeserving destitute could be both arbitrary and a matter of life and death. Perhaps our modern equivalent is 'bed blocking', as health services and local authority social care teams argue over who is responsible for elderly care.

The society of 200 years ago was changing dramatically, and the radically different demographics of rural areas versus new, sprawling urbanisations meant that health care had to be delivered differently – for the less well off, this meant treatment in hospitals rather than at home, in workhouse infirmaries if a family was too poor even for charity. Throughout all this, the wealthy were able to call upon the best doctors, to be seen in the comfort of their own homes, and were likely to be on the Boards that made decisions about what should be done with those less fortunate.

It was ever thus, it seems.

Chapter 1

The structure of the medical profession
1750–1850

In the late eighteenth and early nineteenth centuries, the medical profession was beginning to develop a level of professional feeling that was to lead to a drive for greater status and reform of the structure of medical training. The way a medical man saw his career at the beginning of the nineteenth century was markedly different to the attitudes that existed one hundred years earlier.

Apothecaries had once been viewed as mere tradesmen; their manufacture and dispensing of medicines something that operated from a shop or warehouse rather than a surgery. By the early nineteenth century, they had become recognised as doctors in their own right, rather than simply a servant of the university-trained physician.

The occupation of 'barber-surgeon' disappeared mid-century when the barbers and surgeons parted company and set up individual guilds. No longer was the man who cut your hair also allowed to take your leg off. Specialist surgeons in hospitals were treated with greater respect, if not quite yet as a 'gentleman'.

Those pure physicians, who were generally higher up the social scale and had diagnosed, but not physically treated, illness in their patients (other than by the prescribing of medicines) were now joined by a larger group of practical, well-educated young men who were of sons of the burgeoning middle-classes and had trained in Scotland or on the Continent of Europe. Those who had, in the early eighteenth century, practised medicine in rigidly defined groups were now more likely to be perceived by the public as one professional class.

However, amongst the professionals themselves there was rivalry and suspicion, and for the physicians, a determination that not too many of the 'tradesmen' or craftsmen would climb the professional ladder. Mercifully, by the turn of the nineteenth century, jealousies and petty battles were settling, which could only be good news for the patients, who were always divided into those who could pay the physician's inflated fees and those who could not, with the latter having to consult their local apothecary for medical advice.

In general terms, medical men were still officially divided into three categories before 1815: physicians, surgeons and apothecaries, which aligned with the four categories of medicine – physic, surgery, pharmacy, and midwifery, and there were not the significant number of specialities we would expect to see in the twenty-first century.

Physic was the diagnosis and treatment of internal diseases, by medical (rather than surgical) means. A physician would take a patient's full medical history, as far as it was then understood, including their lifestyle and general constitution. The pulse was taken, the breathing observed and often a disproportionate amount of notice was taken of a patient's urine.

Surgery necessitated the treatment of external disorders, including those of the eye and teeth. Sexually transmitted diseases came within the purview of the surgeon, as did fractures and dislocations, the dressing of ulcers and wounds, and any internal medical problem requiring an incision.

Pharmacy was the domain of the apothecary or druggist who compounded their own medications and preparations and sold them wholesale or over the counter in his own shop.

Midwifery was, in many cases, the traditional domain of the female midwife; throughout history an important assistant and witness to any birth. In the eighteenth century, doctors – then all male – asserted that their skills as 'man-midwives' offered women a safer option.

These branches of medicine were the province of three very distinct groups of medical men.

Physicians

This branch of the profession was ostensibly reserved for the man who had studied at university (abroad, or in Scotland, if he were not an Anglican. At this time those with a non-conformist background were not admitted to university in England) and had obtained a degree in medicine. Those men practising in London were required to be members of the London (later Royal) College of Physicians and were often graduates of Oxford, Cambridge or Trinity College, Dublin, who may not have had any contact with a patient during their training. That training was largely based on studying the writings of Hippocrates and Galen. Their final examination was a thesis defended in Latin – and it was even possible to pay someone else to take this for you.

The physician's main competitor was the surgeon, who, against regulations, may have prescribed medicine to treat a patient and as early as the 1600s, physicians also became impatient with those apothecaries who advised (often poor) patients and prescribed a remedy.

Despite these anomalies, physicians were considered to be the highest branch of medicine, and thus they never undertook to use their hands in manual treatments, rarely touched patients, and would certainly not consider dispensing their own medicines. Their education, supposedly taking in all aspects of surgery and pharmacy as well as physic, gave them the right to oversee the medical work undertaken by a surgeon or apothecary, yet they may have had little experience of patients, other than by observation of their masters in college.

Physicians were generally considered gentlemen, and indeed commentators of the time felt that to be a gentleman was a pre-requisite for the job:

> *The character of a physician ought to be that of a gentleman, which cannot be maintained with dignity, but by a man of literature…If a gentleman, engaged in the practice of physic, be destitute of that degree of preliminary and ornamental learning, which is requisite…if he do but speak on any subject either of history or philosophy, is immediately out of his depth…*[this] *is a real discredit to his profession.*
>
> (Thomas Withers MD Physician to the
> York County Hospital 1774)

There were other physicians who did not belong to the Royal College, however. This was especially true of men who trained and worked outside London. In Scotland, for example, many belonged to other colleges, such as those established in Glasgow in 1599 and Edinburgh in 1681. These men could not become 'Fellows' of the Royal College, as those who attended Oxbridge and Dublin universities could, and therefore had no say in the way their professional body was governed. They were considered of lower status, and some felt them to be subversive, or worse – 'unpatriotic'. This led to disputes within the Royal College itself, as these 'Licentiates' felt that they should qualify as Fellows after a given period of time; many of them had good reputations in London or positions in hospitals. Coming under attack, the Fellows emphasised that in fact, most in their ranks had taken additional lectures in Scotland and abroad, and were regularly seen walking the wards of London hospitals in the position of pupil. Their determination to retain the privilege of an education in Oxbridge and Dublin universities led to charges of un-gentlemanly conduct within the College itself, as Fellows moved to restrict even the most qualified of men on the basis of low birth and their 'democratical and levelling spirit'.

Ultimately, it became clear that the sheer number of licentiates graduating from respected schools of medicine such as Glasgow and Edinburgh highlighted how similar many of the men were in terms of class and education. It was often those trained outside the universities that qualified their members to Fellowship that were responsible for making real discoveries in the field of medicine.

The Royal College of Physicians itself did not have a first membership qualification until 1860, when it then expected and examined on, surgery and midwifery skills in addition to physic.

This was a period when scientific discovery was moving apace, and each new breakthrough increased the public interest across all classes. The study of human anatomy fascinated many, and the examples in this book indicate that by the early 1800s, hospitals and infirmaries across Britain were staffed by men from very different backgrounds to those accepted one hundred years earlier.

Surgeons

The profession of 'Barber-surgeon' developed across medieval Europe and included those willing to perform surgery (unlike other doctors who would not). They were often responsible for treating those injured at war, on land and sea, and would usually learn as an apprentice to an older, more experienced man. In the earliest days, they were often ill-trained and illiterate, but they performed vital services that others often would not, such as taking out teeth, administering enemas, and undertaking amputations. They would, of course, also cut your hair and offer a shave. English barbers and surgeons had created separate guilds until 1540 when Henry VIII merged them into the 'United Barber-Surgeons Company'. Henry's actions had not taken into account the surgeons' belief that they were a profession worthy of greater respect, and in 1745 there was a permanent parting of the ways when King George II established the London College of Surgeons. Barbers were no longer permitted to undertake any surgical procedures other than pulling teeth and bloodletting. The College remained a City Livery Company in order to offer the Freedom of the City to members after they had completed an apprenticeship, but this was undermined when their Examiners ceased to require proof of apprenticeship. The Company of Surgeons had also failed to include anything in the new Act that covered the powers to compel surgeons to serve an apprenticeship, or to take an examination, thus making it weaker than when it was allied with the Barbers. Although the Company of Surgeons had built a new anatomy theatre near Newgate Gaol, in order to remain sufficiently close to the hangman's noose to dissect the bodies of executed criminals in as fresh a condition as possible, in the mid-eighteenth century the standard of teaching there began a decline.

Many surgeons of the period saw their calling as practical rather than academic and thought students were best taught by example rather than by the rigours of a bookish, university education. A surgeon in a hospital or infirmary might agree to take on a number of students to become their assistants and to train under them purely in surgery. These young men paid a premium for the privilege, and others could watch the work whilst paying a lower fee. Those outside the capital didn't always consider it necessary to become a member of the Company, as it did not affect their status or impact on their work. The traditional system was further undermined in 1749 when officers who had been in the services since the accession of George II could take up any trade without serving an apprenticeship. Many of these officers had been saving lives using a form of surgery, albeit it very rough and ready and they refused to be examined by the Company.

Much of the early instruction in surgery was offered by private schools, such as that established by William Hunter, but it was the development of the large hospitals that once again established surgery as a regulated, respected profession, and most of them were launched by public subscription, to ensure treatment and medicine was available to the poorest. At the end of the seventeenth century only St Bartholomew's and St Thomas's, alongside Bethlem (or 'Bedlam') as a specialist hospital for the insane, remained open to patients. However, the Westminster Infirmary was opened in 1720 and by the middle of the eighteenth century, many of the biggest teaching establishments still open in the twenty-first century had been founded, including Guy's in 1721, St Georges in 1734, The London Hospital in 1740, and the Middlesex in 1745. The Edinburgh medical school was founded in 1736, and the London Hospital was taking students by 1742 and was a professionally run teaching hospital within forty years. This rapid expansion continued well into the nineteenth century, with figures suggesting that by 1850 there were around 150 general hospitals nationwide.

Although in England the universities still remained aloof from this practical method of educating surgeons, the Scottish medical schools (along with Trinity College, Dublin) became the best in the country, and in addition to expert tuition could offer examinations and licensing qualifications unavailable to students at English hospitals. A change occurred in 1769 when it was agreed that all practising surgeons should occasionally offer lectures on their subject. This prompted Guy's Hospital to start a course of surgical teaching. Each surgeon could take on up to four students as apprentices or 'dressers' who were, in effect, a surgeon's assistant, caring for and taking responsibility for less serious cases, and although the number of formal apprenticeships went into decline, ambitious pupils were still keen to attach themselves to the best surgeons, often at great expense. For example, when, in 1789, a young man bound himself to Dr William Blizard, a surgeon at The London Hospital and co-founder of the medical school there (mostly at his own expense), he paid £500 for the privilege.

By the early nineteenth century, the teaching of surgeons had become more organised, with less onus on the student himself to ask pertinent questions and more emphasis on the role of the surgeon as a tutor. Reports from the Middlesex Hospital suggest a full itinerary, across six days a week:

8am to 9am – Midwifery

9.30am to 11am – Chemistry or Medicine (alternating)

11am – Demonstrations (Anatomy)

1pm to 2pm – Walking the hospital

2pm to 4pm – Anatomy

6pm to 7.30pm – Physiology

7.30pm to 9pm – Surgery

Twice weekly additional lectures on Materia Medica (that is the body of knowledge about any substance used in healing) were held in the evenings, with optional attendance at Natural Philosophy classes and the weekly Medical Society.

It is important to note here that the change in the way surgery was taught was not universally popular. Some surgeons were concerned that it offered the opportunity for apothecary's apprentices in a country practice to become surgeons in less than a year, and there were doubts as to the efficacy of lectures as a replacement for teaching at a patient's bedside.

On the subject of lectures…we must declare our joint opinions, and they are incontrovertible. If they had been practised and contained principles and rules founded upon judgement and experience, with a

regard to the authority of others as well as their own, they would have been highly useful; if, on the contrary, they have leaned to physiology and experiment, with contempt for all other opinions but their own, they would have been pernicious. The good therefore arising from lectures, unless under certain conditions, must be at least problematical.
(Memorial to the Governors of Middlesex Hospital 1788)

The privately run school of medicine provided education to the greatest number of students during this period. William Hunter, having taken over the school rather than founded it, created one of the most famous schools at Great Windmill Street in 1746, which worked closely with the Middlesex Hospital; private establishments were still at the height of their popularity well into the nineteenth century. They were supported by the Company of Surgeons, and the *Westminster Journal* of 1746 suggests that each night in London there was the opportunity for an enthusiastic pupil to attend one of about five different lectures. Many of these would have included a dissection, and many of the bodies obtained by the notorious 'resurrection men' (see Chapter 3) were 'touted' around these private schools who were always short of material to practice on.

Great teachers, such as William Hunter's brother, John, also created wonderful collections of specimens that, in Hunter's case, are still referred to today at The Hunterian Museum, part of the Royal College of Surgeons.

These rapid developments in the teaching of surgery had left the Company of Surgeons in a difficult position. Modernisation was required, and in 1796 it was decided (despite opposition from members) to apply for a new constitution, and new properties were purchased in the area of Lincoln's Inn Fields in London. At last, after much discussion, in 1800 The Royal College of Surgeons in London was born on presentation of a new Royal Charter. It did not become the Royal College of Surgeons in England until 1843 when Queen Victoria granted a new Royal Charter.

Where the Company of Surgeons had failed to impact on the lives of many provincial surgeons, the Royal College began to impose its new structure on a more effectively regulated and professional section of the medical community.

Apothecaries

The third branch of the medical profession was the apothecary, traditionally somebody who dispensed medicines they had prepared themselves.

The apothecary was often the person to whom the public would turn for advice, especially as they began to diagnose and prescribe as well as make their own medical preparations, but to many, the apothecary was a tradesman rather than of the professional classes. Certainly, apothecaries started off as members of the Company of Grocers, but they had their own Society by 1615 and in that same century began to come into direct conflict with the physicians.

Until the eighteenth century, the role of the apothecary had been very much at the behest of the physician. The apothecary was only allowed to make and dispense medicines as prescribed by a physician; they could not diagnose or treat a patient directly and if they did so they were liable to prosecutions for encroaching on the rights of the physician to be the sole dispenser of physic. However, it became clear that there were many more apothecaries than physicians and that the public, particularly the poor, would regularly turn to them for medical advice, even going as far as to ask them to make home visits, very much the domain of the physician. By the beginning of the eighteenth century, apothecaries outnumbered physicians by ten to one in London and as many, if not more, in provincial towns and villages, and the persistent challenging of physicians culminated in a court case: The Royal College of Physicians v Rose. That case, in its eventual perpetuation of the apothecary's status as a 'purveyor of goods' rather than as a medical man, (despite acknowledging that in practice, he was a regular attendee, offering advice at the sick beds of the poor) has been quoted as having implications for the status of apothecaries and the general practitioner well into the twentieth century.

Apothecaries undertook an apprenticeship, usually of five or seven years, and by the mid-eighteenth century, these apprenticeships were regularly advertised in the local press.

After the apprenticeship ended, the man may supplement his learning with a spell walking the wards of a hospital, taking in dissection (often of corpses obtained by resurrection men), midwifery and further medicine. After the enactment of the Apothecaries Act 1815, the profession was much more closely regulated, and after a mandatory five–year apprenticeship was completed, a student must attend courses in chemistry, Materia Medica and medical botany, two courses in anatomy and physiology, and two on the theory and practice of medicine. Many who had taken these courses also entered themselves for the membership of the Royal College of Surgeons.

In reality, once in practice, there were few who acted as pure physicians or surgeons and a man apprenticed to a surgeon may also practice as an apothecary and vice versa. This gave rise to another frequently described occupation, that of 'surgeon-apothecary', a role that is very much like today's General Practitioner or GP.

Medicine was an over-crowded profession, more so after the end of the Napoleonic wars, when a significant number of ex-naval and military surgeons also wanted to continue their work in civilian life, despite having had only most rudimentary training before joining up. In 1845, around 1,000 entrants for the necessary examinations were licensed to practise, when there were vacancies for half that number.

'Irregular' practitioners

If a doctor was an 'irregular practitioner', then they could have been from one of the many groups who exercised influence outside the 'regular' categories. These men and women provided medical services for centuries – midwives, horse-doctors, chemists, nurses and pedlars, even the village wise-woman – and far from being seen as 'quacks' they were, despite having no formal training, often respected members of a community.

The true 'quack' sold medicine knowing that it wouldn't work. Many medical men considered any alternative treatments to those generally accepted, having no proof of efficacy, were as good as quackery. This labelled many herbalists and chemists alongside those travelling pedlars hawking expensive and useless cure-alls.

The development of professional standards in the nineteenth century

The nineteenth century saw a significant increase in the requirement to pass professional examinations and obtain a licence to practice from relevant Colleges. The Royal College of Surgeons was founded in 1800 and offered the qualification, by examination, of Member of the Royal College of Surgeons (MRCS). After the passing of the Apothecaries Act in 1815, apothecaries needed a licence to practise from the Society of Apothecaries, obtaining the qualification of Licentiate (LSA). The LSA became a comprehensive examination in subjects such as anatomy, physics, chemistry and botany. Students also had to find a placement working in a hospital, infirmary, or dispensary, initially for six months, later increased to a year. These qualifications quickly became the professional 'standard' and by 1840 more than ninety per cent of all newly qualified medical professionals had the letters MRCS LSA after their names.

The Royal College of Physicians took longer to insist on higher standards of education, and it was not until the Medical Act of 1858 that a man had to show a level of knowledge in more than the Classics. Money and a university education could no longer buy you membership of the Royal College, and in 1860 it established the membership examination (MRCP) as the necessary qualification for all new practitioners. In the second half of the nineteenth century, the Scottish colleges of surgery and medicine came together to offer double and triple qualifications, resulting in a long list of letters after a man's name. The 'Triple Qualification' was offered by the Royal College of Physicians, and the Royal College of Surgeons in Edinburgh and the Faculty of Physicians and Surgeons of Glasgow. Practitioners might be listed as 'Lic.R.Coll.Phys.Edin, 1886. Lic.R.Coll.Surg.Edin, 1886. Lic.Fac.Phys. Surg.Glasg, 1886.'

Chapter 2

The great Voluntary Hospital movement

As with many other services we now take for granted, especially when they are provided by the state, the great London hospitals, and many provincial hospitals were actually founded by charitable donation. A hospital is 'voluntary' when it has been provided for the local area by appeal to the public, or occasionally by one keen philanthropist. They are contrasted to the 'royal' or 'endowed' hospitals, some of which had their roots in the monasteries of the time before the Reformation, and which could rely on a source of income other than public appeal. Even when closed, post-Reformation, St Bartholomew's was re-endowed by King Henry VIII, following a petition by the Lord Mayor to ensure there remained a place of safety for the blind, the mentally ill and the chronically sick. The 'endowed' hospitals also include St Thomas's, re-endowed by Edward VI, and Guy's Hospital, built and maintained in perpetuity by the investments of its founder, Thomas Guy.

London was a sick city to live in, and those who were fascinated by medicine were keen to make a difference. The study of medicine and surgery became increasingly popular, and there was soon the recognition that hospitals could be far more than mere refuges. With new treatments being developed for even the most dangerous of diseases, it was an opportunity not to be missed, and the movement brought together great minds to a common purpose.

London was the focus of much of the early investment, and as with many organisations, like minds were drawn together. This explains why so many great general hospitals are close together in central London. The first of the 'new wave' of voluntary hospitals was Westminster Hospital, built in 1720 to address the needs of the local poor. St George's, in Hyde Park, followed in the next decade, and in 1740, The London Hospital was built close to the city going east towards the then village of Mile End. In 1745, the Middlesex Hospital was founded and sited north of the river, serving an area that included Soho. Voluntary hospitals were independent and relied on charitable donations to survive. They were administered by committees of lay people and they, like some of the doctors, would be in voluntary and honorary positions.

Before the end of the first decade of the nineteenth century, London was well served by seven general hospitals, four lying-in hospitals, two for infectious diseases, the Lock Hospital for venereal disease and an eye hospital. At the same time, those in the provinces were not slow to realise the need for similar establishments in their area and in the first part of the eighteenth century the Edinburgh Royal Infirmary, Addenbrookes in Cambridge, and Bristol Royal Infirmary were all founded. The new metropolitan centres soon followed suit and in the second half of the century, Manchester Royal Infirmary, Birmingham General and Glasgow Royal Infirmary all came into being, and further specialist hospitals were built, to treat eye diseases, offer maternity facilities, or a focus on disorders of the ear nose and throat.

Admission to these hospitals was not open to everyone, as the charities founding them often set conditions that they were specifically 'for relieving the sick and needy and other distressed persons'. The London Hospital in Whitechapel stated it was 'for the sick and injured poor of the East End, particularly manufacturers and seamen and their families'. Similarly, the Lock Hospital, opened by William Bromfield in 1747, was specifically founded 'for the treatment of venereal disease'.

It was rare for a hospital to admit contagious diseases, and others would not treat sexually transmitted diseases. Occasionally they would allow admission, but only at the payment of a higher than usual fee. St Bartholomew's, St Thomas's and Guy's accepted fever patients, and only Guy's and the Middlesex admitted 'incurable' patients. Admission usually depended on nomination by a governor or subscriber to the hospital, or a petition, the payment of fees, and a surety against the cost of burial expenses should the patient die.

In many cases, fees were paid by friends and family, or by the parish, though in some cases of extreme need hospitals waived the fees. It was typically expected that patients with a settlement in London should be paid for by their parish. Sureties against the cost of any burial were provided by the parish, employers, a military or naval officer, or by commercial bondsmen, at a price. This is a good place to point out again that the patients in these hospitals were usually poor. Wealthier patients could afford, and preferred, to pay a well-known doctor to attend them at home.

Inevitably, there were many conditions doctors could not treat and many remedies that did not work. However, the hospitals contributed to a general improvement – more babies were registered than burials, and the staff met the obligations of their charitable function by working to take care of a patient's moral state too.

The general standard of medical care in these hospitals was not high, and at times people would find themselves lying in cramped conditions, with the ever-present smells and sounds of other patients. As sometimes still happens today, any infections harboured in the building could spread rapidly, especially if proper antisepsis regimes are not used, as they weren't in this period. So typhus and other dangerous conditions could spread rapidly through crowded wards kept none-too-clean. The staff were not always keen to open the windows – the hospitals were often sited in cramped and dirty parts of the city. But to have cleaned the ward regularly and to admit fresh air would have gone some way to ensure infections didn't spread. Research shows, however, that death rates were not high – around ten per cent, and despite the fact that there were few effective drug treatments; the majority of patients went home rested and cured. This might have been a reflection of the fact that no one with any difficult-to-treat or infectious disease was admitted in the first place.

In some of the hospitals, strict rules were in place to ensure a patient took the time to thank their maker, and have religious instruction. They might also be required to undertake work around the hospital, abstain from alcohol, swearing and behaving or dressing immodestly. Breaching these rules could lead to a patient being discharged, regardless of how far they were from the end of their treatment.

Of course, there were some that, knowing their way around the system, ignored the rules to get the treatment they wanted – telling lies about their sexual behaviour, or the diseases they might have had.

As the patients increasingly became medical specimens for the education of the many students who populated the hospitals in the nineteenth century, they would have found the treatment was 'done to' them, and any thought that they might more successfully treat the whole person, engaging mind and body, was lost in the fervour of learning, and of being part of a fast-moving profession, keen to try out new ideas, whilst ensuring a speedy throughput of patients in what were increasingly busy environments.

Other hospitals were built at this time, outside the voluntary system. Many local and district councils provided the funding to build and staff isolation hospitals, and an examination of the records of asylums for the mentally ill show that they were built and run by the local authority – often being called 'County Asylums'. Poor Law establishments were the medical treatment of last resort for the poorest, who would often rather die than enter the workhouse infirmary.

The voluntary hospital, along with the increasing number of dispensaries, which provided drugs to the poor and dealt with outbreaks of contagious diseases, radically changed the ways in which patients – the poorer ones at least –were treated.

It is remarkable to think that these voluntary hospitals provided the majority of the cutting edge care and treatment development until the 1920s and 1930s when city councils began to take on responsibility for new buildings.

The hospitals at Guy's and St Thomas's are interesting, as the medical education and treatment they offered during the period 1750 to 1850 are illustrative of the great advances made and the medical schools that were established there trained a number of the men whose lives we follow in this book, including the poet John Keats.

Between St Thomas's and Guy's, St Thomas's is much the older of the two hospitals. From its origins in the infirmary of the Augustinian priory St Mary the Virgin, which burned down in 1212, it was rebuilt dedicated to St Thomas of Canterbury in 1215, remaining on that site, just south of London Bridge, for 350 years, until the advent of the railways required it be moved to its current site in Lambeth.

Guy's Hospital was established by Thomas Guy, who was a governor of St Thomas's, a bookseller and publisher who made a considerable amount of money having invested in the South Sea Bubble. It was built close to St Thomas's, in fact just across the road in St Thomas's Street. It was originally designed to be a lunatic asylum, or as a hospital to take in those either refused by its larger neighbour or deemed incurable. However, the demand for emergency and acute services in London was such that it soon became as important as St Thomas's and they became 'United Borough Hospitals' in 1802. They were staffed by highly trained physicians and surgeons whose lectures and tutelage of apprentices and pupils ensured that the United Hospitals could offer one of the most comprehensive medical educations in Great Britain.

St Thomas's medical school maintained specialities in the teaching of surgery and anatomy, whilst Guy's focused on lecturing students on the Materia Medica, botany and medicine. A man might be a surgeon at one hospital and teach in the other, as was the case for Sir Astley Cooper and students would switch between buildings according to the lectures they were attending. This happy co-operation lasted until after Sir Astley Cooper retired from lecturing, although there was some dispute over who should succeed him, and his consequent determination to establish an anatomy school at Guy's to rival that at St Thomas's led to a chill in the relationship.

It was necessary for a student of medicine to observe operations as they took place, and in the *Memorials of Jon Flint South*, a pupil there in 1813, we have a vivid sense of the conditions they were required to study under, and worse still, the horror that awaited the patients who must be exposed to the crowd in an atmosphere where even the healthy could barely breathe.

> *The operating theatre was of utterly inadequate size for the number of pupils who congregated, as the pupils of either hospital had by agreement the right of attending both…The general arrangement of all the theatres was the same. A semi-circular floor and rows of semi-circular standings, rising one above the other to the large skylight which lighted the theatre. On the floor, the surgeon operating, with is dressers, the surgeons and apprentices of both hospitals, and the visitors, stood about the table, upon which the patient lay, and so placed that the best possible view of what was going on was given to all present. The floor was separated by a partition from the rising stand-places, the first two rows of which were occupied by other dressers, and behind a second partition stood the pupils, packed like herrings in a basket, but not so quiet, as those behind were continually pressing on those before often so severely that several could not bear the pressure and were continually struggling to relieve themselves of it, and had not unfrequently to be got out exhausted. There was a continual calling out of 'heads, Heads' to those about the table, whose heads interfered with the sight-seers, with various appellatives… The confusion and crushing was indeed, at all times, very great, especially when an operation of importance was to be performed, and I have often known even the floor so crowded that the surgeon could not operate till it been partially clearer…With all this struggling for the best places, it was very rarely any quarrelling occurred; everyone seemed to consider he must put up with the pushing and squeezing if he could only contrive to get a glimpse of what was going on; but the majority had to draw largely upon their imaginations of what they fancied they saw…*
>
> (Quoted in The Weekes Family Letters by John M.T. Ford)

The apothecary was an important figure in the life of the hospitals, as he was also the resident medical officer responsible for the medical patients, when there were no physicians on duty, and for any prescriptions required by surgical patients. John Ford describes the apothecary's suite of rooms in *The Weekes Letters*, as Hampton Weekes (see Chapter 9) spent a good deal of his time there.

*There was a laboratory where the medicines were made, a shop where
they were dispensed, with store rooms underneath, and as with so many
pharmacies, there was a little room at the back for the apothecary.
Whitfield's was a mere 12½ ft by 7 ft.*

These facilities would be very cramped as Richard Whitfield, the apothecary
at the turn of the nineteenth century and one of a number of Whitfields to
hold the post, had two apprentices and two assistants.

The patient's perspective

On what basis might you be admitted to one of the big London hospitals, or
those set up by charitable foundations in the provinces?

The Lancet described a hospital's functions as to assist 'suitable cases
for charity, supply the wants of the afflicted, and obtain the assistance of
eminent advisers with the comfort of adequate provision, whilst they are
unable because of sickness or accident to follow their normal pursuits'.
(Quote by Geoffrey Rivett from nhshistory.net.)

However, as mentioned previously, the fact that you were poor, and were
sick, did not automatically guarantee you treatment. These were charitable
organisations, but they did not consider themselves under an obligation
to assist those entitled to make an application under the Poor Law, as the
distinction between poor and destitute was relatively clear cut in the eighteenth
and nineteenth century mind. To be poor was to have hope, and charity
would be there to help you when you needed it and put you back in a position
where you would be able to help yourself once more. Their benevolence also
extended to the low-paid workers, who had some small means, but nothing
like enough to pay for their treatment privately. To be destitute, it seems was
almost to be given up for lost. They could neither recover speedily enough, or
when better ensure they could make their way out of poverty without a good
deal more help than was available, so any application they made would be
rejected, as would anyone who looked for treatment for the long haul – having
a chronic complaint requiring months of treatment that would inevitably end
with them becoming a burden on the charity.

These charitable hospitals were there for the 'deserving' poor, and as such
were open to the vagaries of the religious or social beliefs of those making
the decisions. Those considered 'fallen women', or those regularly drunk,
or suffering from a sexually transmitted disease, could find themselves
locked out.

Geoffrey Rivett quotes a well-known hospital administrator called Henry Burdett, who seems to sum this attitude up nicely:

The object of the hospitals is to cure with the smallest number of beds the greatest number of cases in the quickest possible time. The people who are entitled to free relief are those who are able to maintain themselves independently of all extraneous assistance until the hour of sickness when the breadwinner, for instance, is struck down, or the added expense of sickness in the home renders it necessary that the hospital or dispensary should step in.

Chapter 3

Digging for dissection – feeding the horrors of the anatomy table

However depressing the thud of earth on the coffin-lid may be, it is music
compared to the rattle of gravel and thump of spades which heralds a
premature and unreverend resurrection…

Dorothy L Sayers:
The Unpleasantness at the Bellona Club 1928

When discussing the training of doctors in this section, it is impossible to avoid the subject of dissection, and necessary to consider how the bodies found their way to the tables around which keen students would gather, to better understand the workings of the human body.

Satirical cartoons of the period, such as *Death in the Dissecting Room* by Thomas Rowlandson (1757–1827) fed a view common at the time – that doctors were ghoulish, enjoying the desecration of the dead and treating the bodies disrespectfully. Rowlandson's cartoon shows the doctor, and those working with him, conducting multiple dissections, whilst a female body is seen lying pitilessly on the floor in the foreground. A man delivers yet another cadaver and is looking anxiously behind him, as it is certain the body will have been obtained illegally. Skeletons and specimen jars are everywhere, along with other unidentifiable body parts and the instruments used to remove them from the body. Death represented by a skeleton, leaps from a cupboard, aiming a deadly arrow at the doctor in charge.

A legal dilemma

The obtaining of a cadaver for the purposes of dissection had caused considerable hand-wringing in both the legal and medical professions for centuries. As long ago as 1541, the Royal Company of Barbers and Surgeons (the predecessor of the Royal College of Surgeons) lobbied for, and had conferred upon it, a licence to dissect four executed criminals per annum, increased to six by Charles II. This not only offered the first opportunity for a legal supply (albeit a tightly regulated and restricted one) of dead bodies for dissection but also began the perception of dissection as something degrading, perpetrated only on those at the bottom of the social scale. This was the legal position for some 200 years.

In 1752 George II passed what became known as The Murder Act, for 'better Preventing the horrid Crime of Murder'; it offered an additional deterrent to the act of murder: 'the crime of murder has been more frequently perpetrated than formerly…and…it is thereby become necessary that some further terror and peculiar infamy be added to the punishment of death'.

Judges were given the discretion to substitute 'donation for dissection' in place of 'gibbeting in chains'. Both additional punishments, to occur after death, were designed to deny the murderer the comfort of a decent burial. The horror of dissection was thus increased, as the removal of a body to the Royal College of Surgeons – the only official recipient of the cadaver – prevented the felon's family from giving their loved one a Christian burial. Anyone attempting to rescue the bodies of their loved one from this grim fate, which also denied pagan beliefs, was liable to transportation for seven years, with early return also punishable by death. Superstitions about death and the afterlife were rife at this time, and there were frequent gatherings at executions, determined to 'rescue' the body of the dead criminal and ensure the surgeons did not get the chance to take the corpse to pieces. In fact, the riots and threats of revenge were a contributory factor in the decision to end the spectacle of public execution and take the carrying out of the final act within the prison walls. The fear of dissection is closely linked to that of the ultimate punishment introduced by the Tudors, that of hanging, drawing and quartering, which also denied the right to observe custom and practice and offer the chance for redemption in the afterlife; as Ruth Richardson states in *Death, Dissection and the Destitute*:

> *Dissection represented a gross assault upon the integrity and identity of the body and upon the repose of the soul, each of which – in other circumstances – would have been carefully fostered … those who framed the Act appear to have been concerned to a much greater extent with the infliction of punishment than with incidental benefit to science.*

Key figures in the development of the study of anatomy in the eighteenth century are the brothers William and John Hunter. William Hunter thought of the body as useful not only to anatomists but to artists as well. Indeed the flayed corpse of a murderer, still in the Royal Academy collection, was nailed to a cross by sculptor Thomas Banks and painters Benjamin West and

Richard Cosway, to illustrate how far previous artistic depictions of Christ's crucifixion were from anatomically accuracy.

William's younger brother, John Hunter, was to become the more famous in the field of comparative anatomy. His influence is present in the work of other men mentioned in this book, most notably Henry Cline and Astley Cooper, men who trained before the implementation of the Anatomy Act in 1832 and at the forefront of the development of the study of anatomy as vital to a successful medical training.

In 1831, the year before the Anatomy Act, only eleven bodies were released to the Company of Surgeons and were legally available for dissection in London, far too few to meet the need of the anatomy schools, which were growing to meet the needs of men who wanted to train as physicians or apothecaries alongside the practice of surgery. The importance of anatomical study was all the more significant, as the profession was beset by surgeons ill-equipped to pass on their meagre skills to the growing number of medical men training in the period 1750–1850.

If a patient was told they needed surgery, they knew they were in danger of losing their life. Surgery was more a case of hacking off, or out, parts of the body believed to be diseased. There was little finesse, and the surgery was undertaken as quickly as possible to prevent the un-anaesthetised patient dying of shock and blood loss. Postoperative infection was almost certain, as there was no knowledge of the need for cleanliness, antisepsis or antibiotics. For many years, the position of surgeon was offered by means of nepotism and social standing, rather than skill, and, as Ruth Richardson maintains, 'it could be truthfully said that high hospital mortality was the price paid by the poor both for the advancement of scientific surgery, and the advancing social status of surgeons'.

The desperate need for dissection

Dissection has been a means of satisfying human curiosity about the body for millennia. Greek physicians, as early as 200 BC are considered to be the earliest to undertake the systematic dissection of a corpse, but the practice was curtailed by the spread of the Roman Empire, as the dissection of human bodies was outlawed in any part of the world ruled from Rome.

It was not until the Renaissance that anatomy schools were established. Padua in Italy became the centre of the Renaissance and led the world in the opportunities it offered anatomists, who travelled there from Britain to study work that also influenced Leonardo Da Vinci and Andreas Vesalius.

Before the eighteenth century, however, a medical education did not require a physician to study anatomy by practical demonstration. In fact, it was thought a waste of time, offering little in the way of valuable information: 'Tis true it pretends to teach us the use of the parts, but this, if it doth at all, it doth imperfectly and after a gross manner...'

The value of dissection to the study of medicine has been incalculable, however. Medical knowledge in Europe over this period had moved forward rapidly, better understanding the workings of disease from the study of dead bodies, and it was vital that British attitudes change in order to keep pace. The Industrial Revolution created a middle class that was increasingly wealthy and expected the best medical treatment their new money could buy, and doctors maintained that progress could not be made without a better knowledge of anatomy.

The progress made was of greatest use in the treatment of general, and solely male, medical matters. Middle-class women, even under the hands of the most skilled of doctors, were to be treated with a respect that may, in some cases, have meant that the true nature of her illness could not be identified. Doctors were required to examine and treat 'blind', rummaging about under the covers, averting eyes from genitalia and learning to 'feel' for the different vital organs by memory. Dissection also offered the only way in which a medical student could learn how a female body functioned, as no such niceties had to be maintained.

The dissecting room could take medical knowledge forward, but the obtaining of the necessary specimens on which to practise was a dark affair. As Ruth Richardson maintains, the Anatomy Act of 1832, which extended the supply of cadavers by allowing the dissection of the poor, unclaimed, souls who died in the workhouse, effectively made dissection a punishment for poverty. In fact, dissection had been undertaken on those who were poor, and at least nominally unclaimed, for many years. Surgeons working in charitable hospitals, even in an 'honorary' position, could perform what was, ostensibly, a dissection, in front of fee-paying students, simply by taking a post-mortem further than was necessary to establish the cause of death. A student notebook of 1822 shows that most patients, dying in charitable or workhouse hospitals, ended up on the dissecting table. Helen MacDonald in *Human Remains, Dissection and its Histories* says: '...the only patients who died and were not dissected in that city were those with vigilant friends who sat with them until they were taken out of the institution in a coffin...but even then bodies were still in short supply'.

On 4 September 1829, *The Times* published 'A Letter to John Bull on the Dissection of his Body' by one 'Gracchus'. The author of the letter urged the 'absolute necessity' of dissection 'for the attainment of surgical and medical knowledge' and enquired as to the best way to meet the demands of the profession 'without doing violence to popular feelings and prejudices'. Gracchus argues against the proposal made by parliament (eventually adopted in the 1832 Anatomy Act) that unclaimed bodies of the poor should be given up for dissection, stating that 'this alternative has something very horrible on the face of it to any man who feels and reverences the spirit of the English constitution'. It would result in a 'stigma on poverty', an 'injustice' and he asked 'do the dying and friendless poor feel nothing?'

The Times responded with vigour:

> *We confess we cannot perceive the injustice of the plan. Where is the injustice in using an unclaimed body for purposes intimately connected with the general good, any more that appropriating unclaimed property to the public service.*

This statement, whilst making the corpses of poor men, women and children sound like little more than forgotten umbrellas, was just the beginning of the paper's objections to Gracchus's view. The paper claimed that it was the poor who undoubtedly suffered the most from inferior surgical techniques, so they surely had a vested interest in the proposal? It quite openly admitted that this provision would not affect the rich, as they were never to be found unclaimed in workhouses, but the piece did not mention that any medical discoveries made would benefit the rich first.

Addressing the poor's apparent pre-death fear of dissection, the paper said:

> *With respect to the supposed feelings of the sick and friendless poor at the prospect of dissection [despite the known fears even of the worst criminals] we are far from thinking with GRACCHUS that they would be very acute. Actual bodily pain and suffering leave little room for the intrusion of ideas connected with other matters; and we doubt exceedingly whether the dread of death would be much augmented by the fear of dissection...*

There was also the suggestion made, that the fear of dissection might dissuade the needy from attending hospital when treatment was necessary, but *The Times* countered that argument:

We question whether the adoption of a regulation, by which the bodies of all persons dying in hospitals and unclaimed for burial by surviving friends and relatives should be declared liable for dissection, would deprive the hospitals of a single patient. The sick poor, like all other sick people, hope to recover, and go into hospital, not to die, but to live. We are aware we must die, but not now, this time we expect to escape. The dying seldom know they are dying and the apprehension of dissection will not disturb those who turn their backs on death…

The Times, like Gracchus, agrees that another proposal – to legalise the sale of bodies by relatives and friends – is a step too far, but seemingly only because the 'lower ranks of life' where, the editor suggests, 'it could only ever operate', would face 'a strong temptation to culpable negligence and inattention in cases of illness if not a bounty upon murder…'

Another idea offered by Gracchus – that 'it shall not be lawful to inter… the body of any man or male child…until the said body shall have been opened by a Physician, Surgeon or Apothecary', and that it would be an offence in law to do otherwise – is dismissed as increasing the public outcry rather than avoiding it, as Gracchus maintains, and the unclaimed poor would still suffer. It would also overwhelm all the practising medical men in the country:

…what a needless and profligate waste of subjects…God help the physician or surgeon who has an extensive practice…his surgery will be converted into a shambles and the ghosts of deceased patients, whom, according to the tale, surround the doors of the doctors by whom they died, will be outnumbered by the multitude of dead bodies; so that a Christian man shall not be able to pick his steps between them to the threshold of the slaughter-house…

The paper points out that Gracchus states his desire to 'familiarize the public with dissection', in order to reduce their fear of it. This will not do: 'We beg GRACCHUS's pardon, but we must say the public desires to be familiarized with no such thing…' *The Times*, in that assertion at least, was probably correct.

The heated arguments on both sides had been continuing for some time and across the nation. A year before the intervention of Gracchus and *The Times*, a fascinating, and scathing, letter had been sent to the *Berkshire Chronicle* and was published on 12 April 1828. Christopher Macure MD wrote:

The gentlemen of 'the profession' are now making a tremendous uproar about the impropriety of punishing body snatchers and the lack of wisdom in our laws for not directing that all persons who die in hospitals and gaols shall be dissected…I think it would be quite as sane were a prospective enactment passed, ordering the bodies of paupers and healthy felons to be cut up and sold in the public market for food… for…it is high time to adopt some mode or other for the more efficient provision of sustenance for a redundant population.

He continued:

But..it is 'the profession' [politicians] with whom I have to deal; and as they are so excessively and gratuitously liberal in disposing of the carcasses of others, I would propose that the Marquis of Lansdowne, Brougham, Hume… and any other thorough-paced patriot, introduce a bill to the legislature, enacting…that every medical student, on being articled, shall give a bond, with securities of 500l that after death, his body be dissected for the benefit and example of the public, unless indeed, he would prefer that operation taking place when alive; but…very few will be agreeable to such an arrangement, the age for dissecting alive will be fixed for 65 years and this will accomplish another great good, …for the operate will become the willing victim of a scientific pursuit! …it should be further enacted that all persons hereafter to be made Peers for the realm, and all persons elected to serve in Parliament, … shall by deed indented, transfer their bodies also after death, to some hospital or school of anatomy in London or Westminster, there to be dissected but with this additional provision, that all the bones of Noble and Hon. Legislators …be subsequently made into skeletons, hung up in Westminster Hall, and properly labelled. Thus will their relics be made to live in the recollection of posterity; and as the wind rushes through the portals of the Hall, the very 'shaking of the dry bones' will serve to raise up a spirit of patriotism and national devotion in their successors…

There were many other letters published in the press to a similar effect, some suggesting that if only the royal family were to agree to be dissected then ALL the country would sign up with them.

The hypocrisy of the ruling classes, who seemed quite happy to allow the bodies of the poor to be pulled apart in the name of science, was regularly noted in the press, especially when any case of body snatching came to the public's notice. Even after the Anatomy Act came into force, the demands of the dissection room regularly outstripped the supply of the unwanted poor, and although much reduced, body snatching was to continue into the twentieth century. In 1839 an anonymous letter was sent to the *Perthshire Chronicle* (11 April) expressing the feelings of many who found the whole idea of dissection abhorrent. The author expressed his horror at the extent of theft and murder to provide bodies for the dissecting room, but that despite society's repugnance, they had only themselves to blame for not crying out 'at the horrors of the practises of medical men':

> *It may seem paradoxical that the author should call in question the sensitiveness of the public on the matter when the papers teem with instances of the anxiety with which the remains of the dead are watched, so often accompanied by desperate resistance to the night robber. But…the care and watchfulness arise, not from any feeling that the wretches who prowl about the abodes of the departed are meditating anything in itself wrong…but because it is a thing which all would wish to prevent when the bodies of their own relatives are in jeopardy, but which they care very little about when the offence is not likely to affect their own families or friends…*
>
> *Who is there, even among those hardened as they are, who practice at the tables in these* [dissecting] *rooms, whose feelings are so blunted as they would expose the bodies of their own friends to the same treatment? Not one…But I shall be told, in the cant of these enlightened days, that these and all similar feelings are mere prejudices… If they be but prejudices, why do not medical men give the bodies of their wives, their sons and their daughters to their students…Why not bring the body to the dissecting room and say "Here behold exposed before you that body which when alive I would not that the winds of heaven should have visited too rudely! Here, take this arm to your closet and admire its symmetry even in death"?…*

The Anatomy Act 1832

It is remarkable to think that an Act, originally drafted to thwart the activities of the body snatchers or resurrection men and to provide an official source of human bodies upon which a surgeon or student of medicine could undertake research, remained in force until 2004, when it was at last replaced by the Human Tissue Act of 2004.

The Anatomy Act 1832 was passed at a time when newspapers were focusing on an outbreak of cholera and on parliamentary reform. So, as in the twenty-first century, contentious legislation could be passed with barely a flutter of interest from the newspapers. The Act gave the hospital medical schools and private schools of anatomy an official means of access to the bodies they required for research and learning. The bodies of lunatics and paupers, those left in workhouses and hospitals with apparently no one to mourn them or pay for a funeral, could be bought from the Poor Law Unions and from those owning eligible institutions, for the purposes of medical research. There was significant opposition to the Bill, as it appeared to make a crime out of dying poor and alone, and deprived a person of their right to a burial in their parish. A death in a workhouse, for example, would, if no one came to collect the body within seven days with the means to pay for a decent funeral, be recorded in the parish register and taken to the medical schools without any act of burial taking place. This provision goes some way towards explaining the particular dread many had of the workhouse as, in addition to separation from family, harsh conditions and the stigma, there was also now the fear of dissection after death, something only previously allowed on the bodies of convicted criminals.

A debate in the House of Commons on 11 June 1844 stated that between 1839 and 1841, the bodies of around 300 paupers had been taken under the provisions of the Act, but it was clear this was still not enough to satisfy the medical fraternity, who needed at least double that number. It was also clear that some masters of a workhouse were not always putting the fee for the body into the coffers for the benefit of all, but pocketing it for themselves. There was also, it seems, a trade in the unwanted and unused parts of the body that could provide a lucrative extra for hospital lecturers. The Act, in that respect, did not end the abhorrent trade of the resurrection men; it simply changed the nature of the profiteer.

The horrors of the dissecting room

For many, the horrors of the dissecting room disgust and intrigue in equal measure. For young doctors, their first terrifying experience of the dissecting room gradually fades as their continued work inures them to the subject as a person, the flesh and organs under their scalpel simply there to give them the opportunity to learn, first hand, the wonderful workings of the human machine. For many, however, that loss of a natural response to death and human bodies was one that awakened in them the sense that they were about to lose something precious, which they resisted, and which persuaded them medicine was not for them.

Hector Berlioz, the nineteenth-century composer, originally intended to be a doctor and was sent to study medicine in Paris in 1821. His situation is not so different from that facing the poet John Keats, or any young man training to be a surgeon-apothecary in the early years of the nineteenth century. His experience of the dissecting room convinced him that his life should be spent in the creative arts, rather than the wards and operating theatres of the big cities. In his memoirs, Berlioz offers a graphic description of his first experience of the hospital dissection room:

> *When I entered that fearful human charnel house, littered with fragments of limbs, and saw the ghastly faces and cloven heads, the bloody cesspools in which we stood, with its reeking atmosphere, the swarms of sparrows fighting for scrapings and rats in the corners gnawing bleeding vertebrae, such a feeling of horror possessed me that I leapt out of the window, and fled home as though Death and all his hideous crew were at my heels.*

This description sounds terrifying enough and in France, more 'fresh' bodies were made available for dissection, officially, than in Great Britain, where access to bodies was restricted; as previously mentioned, the Royal College of Surgeons had since the mid-sixteenth century only been able to dissect the bodies of four felons annually.

In *Digging up the Dead: Uncovering the life and times of an extraordinary surgeon*, author Druin Burch offers a vivid description of the dissecting room at St Thomas's Hospital in the Borough, an area of London already sufficiently putrid to turn a man's stomach.

> *The western wall of the room was covered with glass cases displaying previous dissections, bobbing up and down in their liquid baths if they were muscle, skin and fat, or held up and articulated by pins and wires if they were bone. Other glass cases were scattered around the walls and shelves wherever there was room for them. Under the windows was a large sink for the students to wash their hands. They could also wash the hands of their subjects – or whatever part they were currently investigating. It was the place for disposing of the most liquid bits of the corpses, for washing the faeces and the last meals from within pieces of bowel, or stomach.*

Bodies were laid out on the ten or twelve dissection tables in the room, in various states of decay depending on the swiftness with which they were removed from the churchyard after burial and the success, or otherwise, of the process of pickling in alcohol.

There would be at least six students per corpse, so the room was rapidly filling up. The uncle of the famous doctor William Osler describes the scene thus:

On entering the room, the stink was most abominable. About 20 chaps were at work, carving limbs and bodies, in all stages of putrefaction, and of all colours; black, green, yellow or blue, while the pupils carved them apparently, with as much pleasure, as they would carve their dinners. One was pouring Terebinth on his subject, and amused himself with striking with his scalpel at the maggots, as they issued from their retreats.

That maggot-stabbing student was taking greater risks than he might have realised in his amusing pastime. Burch points out how dangerous the whole scene could be, as personal hygiene, and the putrefaction of the bodies, meant that infection could almost be felt in the atmosphere of the room, ready to strike an unwary student who might accidentally stab themselves with a scalpel, or a simple splinter of bone from a rotting corpse. There were no antibiotics with which to treat any ensuing infection, and should a man succumb, the death could be swift and painful.

The room would also be stiflingly hot, as to open the windows would let in an even greater number of flies, and the stink of the living flesh that gathered in the slum-ridden streets of the Borough. There was a great fire burning at one end of the room, heating a copper pan in which would be placed the bones of a specimen which required a more hasty removal of flesh, or those frustratingly sticky, greasy pieces of fat and tissue that the scalpel was unable to reach. The smells would linger and cling to the clothes of the men in the room, mingling with the sweat of their bodies as they worked for hours in a dangerous miasma.

Strangely, the dissecting rooms of both hospital and private school of anatomy were often treated as an informal 'common room', partly because of the length of time students spent there. Smoking was permitted, as was the consumption of alcohol, and gossip was rife. Games of chess were completed amongst the corpses and although these students may have been glad of the diversion from the horror that surrounded them, others were disgusted by the nature of the conversations and the apparent irreverence shown to the dead.

Aesculapius, in *A Hospital Pupils' Guide*, written as a textbook for students in the first quarter of the nineteenth century described the study of anatomy as 'a beautiful but seductive science', but acknowledged that, rather than encouraging the medical students to examine a corpse and see in it evidence of the workings of a supreme being, it did nothing to discourage a general tendency towards atheism among the young when studying medicine.

In 1823, one Reverend Rennell published his *Remarks on Scepticism*, in which he maintained that the medical student, rather than recoiling in horror at the sight of the corpses, and perhaps treating them with irreverence to cover their discomfort, was 'overpowered with a feeling of indescribable admiration and awe' and saw in the human body the 'immediate work and wisdom of God'. He was concerned, however, that the frequency with which the student is faced with the sight of men laid bare tended towards a hardening of attitude leading to these 'spectacles of mortality' losing their impact and becoming 'matters of course'.

The apparently rowdy behaviour of some students gave commentators of the period opportunity to make class distinctions between the students, suggesting that if a man were sufficiently well educated, and as a 'gentleman' was by definition a 'man of feeling', then the due reverence necessary would be a natural response, despite any initial disgust. Those exhibiting the coarseness, that so worried observers, were by implication of the lower orders.

Dissection became a central part of a medical student's training, and increasingly, whole days might be devoted to it. The memoirs of eminent surgeons suggest that it was a subject that could take over a student's life. Royston Lambert, in his biography of Sir John Simon, recounts:

> *So keen were his anatomical interests that his specimens and instruments overflowed into the cupboard where he kept his food, with the result that, one morning in April 1835, he woke up to find that he had caught (doubtless from infected food) severe erysipelas of the face and head*

So Berlioz's response is unsurprising. The academic term at teaching hospitals in the eighteenth and nineteenth centuries ran from October until May, partly in order to ensure the bodies obtained for teaching purposes did not rot too quickly in the heat of the summer months.

A 'horrid traffic'

'If the horrid traffic in human flesh be not, by some means or other, prevented, the churchyards will not be secure against the shovel of the midnight plunderer, nor the public against the dagger of the midnight assassin.' (Lancet 1829 quoted in Ruth Richardson, *Death Disease and the Destitute.*)

An obscure principle in law, 'nullius in bonis', or the body is the property of no one, was recognised, leading to the presumption that 'there is no property in a corpse', thus making it impossible to steal.

The precedent was set, in 1788, by a case against one Lynn, who was charged with 'disinterring a corpse for the purposes of dissection', although the court would still not consider it a theft per se. It was seen as criminal only because it was 'indecent' and although an offence in law, it was apparently a minor one punishable by a fine or a short term of imprisonment. There is little wonder that the trade continued, and led to the practice of making sure that only the body – not the shroud or any other possession attached to the body, which would have been a theft – was taken from the grave.

In the earliest days, it might be the medical students themselves who resorted to finding their own specimens. The requirement to know the anatomy of the body made dissection a vital component of any course of study. James Blake Bailey, in 1896, wrote an account of *The Resurrection Men in London* to accompany *The Diary of a Resurrectionist, 1811-1812*, a transcription of entries in the handwritten records of Joseph Naples, London 'Resurrection Man' and procurer of bodies for the anatomy lectures, an original diary now held in the archives of the Hunterian Museum in London. He reported that surgeons were concerned that they could be 'punished in one Court for want of skill, and in another Court, the same individual might also be punished for trying to obtain that skill'. In 1828, before the Anatomy Committee, the eminent surgeon Astley Cooper highlighted the story of one young student, rejected by the College of Surgeons 'on account of his ignorance of the parts of the body'. It was revealed that he was a very diligent student, who had failed simply because he was unable, or unwilling, to procure a body for dissection.

The number of corpses required to meet the needs of the students and surgeons is hard to gauge, as it is not known with any certainty how many dead bodies per student was seen as sufficient at the time. Ruth Richardson suggests that when discussion on the subject was at its height in the 1820s and 1830s, the numbers quoted from one, perhaps in pieces, to three whole bodies per student over the course of his training. Richardson highlights figures from the returns of students and corpses made by twelve London anatomy schools in 1826 for the 1828 Select Committee on Anatomy. These show that 592 bodies were dissected by 701 students. Although this supply is far in excess of what could be obtained legally, it is still less than one body per student.

Clearly, there was a market for the bodies of the dearly departed, and thus 'body snatching' became an opportunity for those sufficiently entrepreneurial, and strong of stomach, to make a very good, if far from respectable, living.

Depictions of the resurrection man or body snatcher were regularly to be found in fiction of the time, and the press could make it difficult to tell real life from fantasy, as sensational facts fascinated readers. Bailey found a tale recounted in the *Monthly Magazine* for April 1827 in which students pressurise a sailor, newly returned to England after a long voyage, and on his way to meet his sweetheart, to find them a body for the purposes of dissection. Having disinterred a body as required, the sailor emptied his sack in front of the students, only to find he had dug up his lover, whose death he had been unaware of. Blake compares this to the following real life case:

> *There is a case on record of a child who had died of scrofula, and whose body was brought to St Thomas' Hospital by Holliss, a well-known resurrectionist. The body was at once recognised by one of the students as that of his sister's child; on this being made known to the authorities at the hospital, the corpse was immediately buried before any dissection had taken place*

The cases of Burke and Hare in Edinburgh, and of Bishop and Williams in London, have been written about in some detail, and fictionalised and discussed to the point that they can be seen as terrifying icons of the times they were living in. There were cases where the demand for bodies so outstripped supply that a man might commit murder to provide his client with the best possible specimen, but it was a risk few would take. Most body snatchers were working men who saw their trade as one of demand and supply. Of particular interest here is Joseph Naples, one of the many body snatchers in London in the early part of the nineteenth century. He is believed to be the author of the diary held in the Library of the Royal College of Surgeons, his own personal, contemporaneous record of his transactions in the year between November 1811 and December 1812. It is the only written source we have by anyone working in the trade. It is a diary of few words, but it tells us a great deal about the arrangements and general day-to-day trade of a jobbing body snatcher.

The diary shows that Naples and his team traded in corpses with all the biggest anatomy schools in London, and had opportunities to send cadavers as far as Edinburgh and, in the author's words, 'to the country'. Individual doctors, such as Sir Henry Cline, are named, and St Thomas's Hospital benefits from the delivery of two bodies during this period.

Made redundant by the introduction of the Anatomy Act in 1832, Naples was sufficiently well respected by the men to whom he had supplied bodies that he was offered employment as a servant in the dissecting rooms of St Thomas's Hospital.

Body snatching was clearly not a job taken on for the enjoyment it offered. It was risky – men could be attacked by dogs, or by the increasingly vigilant members of the public determined to thwart them. Many journeys were wasted, perhaps because the graves were guarded, or because the eventual prize was in an advanced state of putrefaction. Sometimes a sexton, primed beforehand with a bribe, simply didn't turn up to grant access.

Body snatchers did not always have to resort to digging. Stooges, often women, were sent into workhouses to act as a grieving relative and steal a body that the authorities saw only as a burden. Mortuaries or 'dead-houses' were few, but body snatchers could take advantage of lax security. Astley Cooper was one of the most successful surgeons of his day and no less able in his dealings with the resurrectionist. He is known to have obtained more, and probably paid the least for, bodies of all varieties, obtained by a group of men with whom he dealt on a regular basis. Yet he thought nothing of them beyond their skill at unearthing fresh subjects. He considered them the lowest of the low, but his disparagement belies the fact that without them, he would not have been able to achieve his rapid rise to fame as a surgeon and lecturer.

It was a filthy trade, which men often found their way into on their return home from the French and Peninsula campaigns, where they had extracted the teeth from the dead on the battlefield to sell for the making of dentures. Once home, they would continue this trade when, having dug up a fresh body, they would remove the teeth to sell separately.

However miserable, it was a potentially lucrative trade, although Naples's diary suggests that once the fees had been shared amongst gang members, and any bribes paid, the income was modest rather than excessive. Compared to the wage of a working man at the time, however, the possibilities were worth the potential risks and the men probably charged the surgeons a premium to cover the hazards involved. They also drafted documents that were a form of blackmail to ensure that, if arrested, the connections to the reputable anatomy schools were discovered, and the men taking advantage of the trade asked to help with bail to avoid the bad publicity. Sarah Wise, in *The Italian Boy: Murder and Grave Robbery in 1830s London* quotes Sir Astley Cooper's accounts for 1818:

'His personal accounts for 1818 show that he paid £14 7s as bail for one of his main suppliers, – a man called Vaughan; 6s to Vaughan's wife; and £13 on "gaol comforts" – food drink and tobacco – for Vaughan when he was imprisoned.'

In the 1820s, as public awareness and opposition grew, the costs to the men desperate to study the intricacies of the human body inevitably rose.

Thwarting the resurrection men.

Whatever the possessors of the practical insensibility, acquired in the dissecting room, may assert to the contrary, we hold it, with the greater part of the community, to be at once a formidable and lamentable evil, that a parent cannot commit its offspring, nor the offspring its parent, to the earth, without the distressing suspicion intruding itself upon the mind, that in a few hours one or the other may be torn from its last resting place, and made an object of traffic among a band of ruffians
Lancet editorial 1829, in Ruth Richardson

The illegal exhumation of a newly buried body was a constant source of worry to the bereaved, who might employ 'protection' of their loved one's graves for a number of days after death, only to find that eventually even bodies in a serious state of decomposition were acceptable for the desperate medical student.

The surgeons themselves were part of the illegal trade. Many, like Sir Astley Cooper, were mentioned by the poet Thomas Hood, who wrote a piece that treats the subject in a light-hearted manner, but at its heart has the truth:

Mary's Ghost by Thomas Hood

'Twas in the middle of the night,
To sleep young William tried,
When Mary's ghost came stealing in,
And stood at his bed-side.

O William dear! O William dear!
My rest eternal ceases;
Alas! my everlasting peace
Is broken into pieces.

I thought the last of all my cares
Would end with my last minute;
But tho I went to my long home
I didn't stay long in it.

The body-snatchers they have come,
And made a snatch at me;
It's very hard them kind of men
Won't let a body be!

You thought that I was buried deep
Quite decent like and chary,
But from her grave in Mary-bone
They've come and boned your Mary.

The arm that used to take your arm
Is took to Dr. Vyse;
And both my legs are gone to walk
The hospital at Guy's.

I vow'd that you should have my hand,
But fate gives us denial;
You'll find it there, at Dr. Bell's
In spirits and a phial.

As for my feet, the little feet
You used to call so pretty,
There's one, I know, in Bedford Row,
The t'other's in the city.

I can't tell where my head is gone,
But Doctor Carpue can:
As for my trunk, it's all pack'd up
To go by Pickford's van.

I wished you'd go to Mr. P.
And save me such a ride;
I don't half like the outside place,
They've took for my inside.

The cock it crows – I must begone!
My William we must part!
But I'll be yours in death, altho'
Sir Astley has my heart.

Don't go to weep upon my grave,
And think that there I be;
They haven't left an atom there
Of my anatomie.

The population of urban areas was growing so significantly during this period that the traditional churchyards were, literally, filled to overflowing. At a burial, the digging of a hole for one body may reveal another, in a further state of decomposition, only just beneath the surface. These were most likely burials of the poor; respectable artisans, trades, and the aspirational working class might be able to afford a deeper plot in a quieter part of the churchyard, or more safely out of town.

Coffins became ever more expensive in order to thwart the resurrectionists, who would find a heavy wooden coffin double- or triple-lined with lead, preventing easy access and making it less likely that a swift exit from the scene of the crime was possible. Those with even larger sums of money would have a vault or a mausoleum built to house the dead of the family, but when it became apparent that those in a position of trust at a graveyard – such as sextons, grave-diggers, and even landowners, could be corrupt and in the pay of the body snatchers, or even agents of surgeons themselves, no one felt safe. This offered opportunities to those eager to bring a new protective option to market. In 1818 the first patent metal coffin was designed specifically to prevent the body snatchers gaining access. Made of cast or wrought iron, it could not be levered apart and its protection could be extended by the means of bars attached to head and footstones, or by digging a tomb that extended for some distance underground. In Scotland, the 'mortsafe' was developed, consisting of an iron cage, or grid of metal, which encased the coffin and was cemented into the ground. For the less well-off something similar could be hired, and maintained until such time as it was believed the body snatchers would think the body was past use. 'Dead-houses' performed the same function, storing a body safely until sufficient decomposition would have taken place.

For the poor, the most successful approach was to act as a community, protecting the churchyards with watch-houses, or using lights to deter the opportunistic thief. The greatest challenge in these situations was becoming wise to the cunning of the resurrection men, gangs of whom would 'case' a parish by asking, often in the pubs, whether anyone had died recently, or laying watch for the passing of a cortège.

Some local history societies have made detailed studies of the churchyards within their area, and reveal good examples of community action to protect the dead of the parish. One such case is that of the 'Streatham Grave Robbers', three men called Lane, Watts and Butler. This story is summarised from a book, *The Streatham Grave Robbers: A Tale of Attempted Body Snatching at Streatham in 1814* by John W Brown.

It was February 1814, and the demand for fresh bodies for the dissecting table was growing to the point that gangs of resurrection men were searching further out of city centres in search of bodies to meet the requirements of the anatomy schools. One night, Thomas Watts entered the churchyard of St Leonard's Church, a prominent parish church in Streatham, on the main route from London to Brighton, and started to dig the newly turned earth on the top of a recently filled plot. Despite doing his best to conceal his actions he was spotted by a vigilant local resident, who, despite the late hour, ran to the nearby White Lion Inn, a prominent stop on the coach route to the coast. There he found a group of late drinkers, who, although the worse for a few tankards of ale, heard the tale with horror and hurried off to the churchyard to catch the body snatcher in the act.

Watts, meanwhile, was finding the compacted earth beneath the topsoil hard to breach and was stopping frequently to mop his brow. As he took a breath, he heard the sound of the heavy-footed vigilantes from the White Lion, attempting to creep up on him and thought it best to flee the scene empty handed, even leaving his shovel behind in a desperate bid to escape over the wall and into the dark countryside beyond the church.

The gang pursuing him saw Watts's escape and were determined to catch him, and it didn't take them long to bring the terrified man to the ground. Not the most loyal of men, he quickly tried to improve his position by giving himself up and naming his co-conspirators. Whilst Watts was digging in the churchyard, one Thomas Butler, a dentist from Southwark, was drinking in another pub, the Red Lion on Streatham Hill, and he was quickly identified

as one of the wanted men and dragged away ignominiously to join his friend
Watts in the local lock-up, guarded by seven Streatham men. William Lane
(also known as Harnott or Arnott), the final member of the gang was also
caught and he too spent the night under lock and key.

The magistrates decided that despite there being no successful snatch,
the men should be committed for trial and some time later, in 1815 they
were all found guilty of 'having unlawfully entered the churchyard of the
Parish of Streatham with the intent to take away the dead body of a certain
person named James Burton there buried'. Burton would have been a
valuable prize; at just 35 years of age, a surgeon would have paid well for his
relative youth. After this incident, the parish had to expend significant sums
to protect newly dug graves from further attack. This cost £11 18s 9d in
1829, and in 1831 the parish spent the then enormous sum of £500 for the
erection of tall railings around the whole area of the churchyard. Ironically
this expenditure would not have been necessary just a year later with the
passing of the Anatomy Act.

Watts, Lane and Butler were sent to prison for three months, this despite
the ineffectual nature of the sortie and the fact that Watts's actions were
sufficient to incriminate all three men. The action of the local community had
resulted not only in the protection of one of their own, but in the conviction
of three men determined to make money from the trade in human misery.

Another case highlights the sheer bravado of the resurrection men. In
November 1829 the *Oxford and City Herald* reported a 'Body snatching
extraordinary':

*On Sat. afternoon, an elderly man, named Curtis, many years known
in Smithfield Market, and who had been for a considerable time ailing,
died at his lodgings in Barbican Court, Barbican. In the course of the
evening two men, dressed in shabby black, and having the appearance
of undertaker's men, brought a shell to the house, and saying they
had come for the old man, were shown into his late apartment, and in
quite a business-like way placed the body in the shell, which they also
carefully removed downstairs and outside the door. Just as they were in
the act of shouldering it, other men in black, and a second shell, were
seen advancing up the court, one of whom asked whose body had they
got there? Instead of any answer from the two first comers, to drop the
shell and corpse on the stairs, and effect their escape was the work of a
moment; but in their flight one of them was recognised as a notorious
resurrectionist. The undertaker's men for such in reality were the latter*

comers, then removed the body in the shell in which it was left which was subsequently ascertained to have been borrowed in the afternoon... and a deposit of 10s left upon it by a strange man...

In Drogheda, close to Dublin, one year later, the *Drogheda Journal* reported a 'Daring outrage of resurrectionists':

On Friday evening, about six o' clock, a party of resurrectionists rushed suddenly into a house in Bow-lane where the corpse of an aged female, named Carroll, was being waked by her friends and neighbours in an upper apartment, and succeeded in possessing themselves of the body which they bore off, before the persons present could offer any effectual resistance. The ruffians acted with the most revolting indecency, dragging the corpse, in its death close, after them through the mud in the street, and unfortunately baffled all in pursuit...

The significance of these cases is how brazen the men were, not just to snatch bodies away from a wake under the noses of mourners, but did so in the full knowledge that they were so well known they were likely to be recognised.

As the men became more desperate, there was an increasing willingness to resort to violence in order to achieve their ends. *The Dublin Evening Packet & Correspondent* of February 1830 reported:

On Monday night, as a man named Albert Neagles, a French man, in the employment of Mr Henry, at Island Bridge, he was on his way home from the manufactuary, he was met by about 16 men, armed with swords and firearms, and who had with them a cart filled with dead bodies, which had been taken out of the Hospital Fields. Five of the resurrectionists followed Neagles and the man in his company, and one of those fellows presented a pistol at Neagles's breast which he pushed aside and another ruffian then struck at Neagles with a sword, cut his hat and wounded his head – One of the resurrectionists called out 'stick him Tom' and another exclaimed 'cut him to pieces Murphy'.

Neagles's companion fled and the resurrectionists left, two of them being arrested in a public house later. Neagles was left bleeding, but survived. He had fought with Napoleon's army and said later that if he had had a sword he would have mowed them down 'like so many cabbage stalks...'

Chapter 4

The rise of the General Practitioner

As this book suggests, the key feature of Georgian and early Victorian medicine is the structure and standing of the profession. It appears, on the face of it at least, to be one of great variety, although it could be argued that to the layperson in the twenty-first century the structure and management of the NHS is at least as confusing. There are still physicians and surgeons, and also GPs, nurse practitioners and specialists, as well as junior doctors, and nurses, staff in training, and all the necessary support staff.

However, the period 1750 to 1850 is a key period in the early development of the medical system we enjoy now, with a general practitioner (GP) as our first point of contact, situated within our local community. There was much shuffling for space, for recognition and for independence; from this time come our consultants and our GPs.

The *Medical and Physical Journal* of 1809 first refers to a 'general practitioner of medicine' and in 1813 elaborated on the description, stating that a GP was a 'general practitioner in medicine surgery and midwifery in which the apothecary would be included'.

The term GP came into common usage between 1810 and 1830, although before that medical practitioners in towns and villages were often still designated as surgeon or apothecary.

The 'Rose' case of 1704 (see Chapter 1) had resulted in the regulation of a position that had already been common in many areas. Despite the hostility of physicians to the idea, Rose permitted those who were dispensing drugs to dispense medical advice as well and thus the apothecary became the medical man of first resort, particularly for those who could not afford expensive physicians fees. Roles merged as the training developed and, without the necessity of a university degree, a man specialising in surgery would also attend lectures in medicine, and an apothecary attend surgical demonstrations. The great surgeon of the day would need to exhibit accuracy in his prescriptions and although the physician might hold the highest social status, it was the surgeon-apothecary who was more likely to have the practical hands-on patient experience necessary to remedy the increasing number of identifiable and treatable conditions. The social status was important, however, and many considered working as an apothecary to be a trade rather than a profession.

Once doctors, or surgeon-apothecaries, began to charge for their service rather than simply the medicines they dispensed, their status depended on how they required their bills to be settled. Practitioners requiring swift settlement in cash, rather than payment by annual account, had a lower social standing, although this more 'lowly' position was often as a result of the generosity of the doctor towards his community; cash payers often being the poorest patients.

Similarly, those who worked for Friendly Societies or attended workhouses were unlikely to be considered 'gentlemen'. Men could struggle to make a living, whilst others, working only for wealthy clients, were received into polite society; although, at the very top, even narrower distinctions were made. In 1890, Lady Warwick pointed out that 'doctors and solicitors might be invited to garden parties, though never, of course, to lunch or dinner'.

When looking at the lives of the men detailed in Chapters 7 and 8 it is clear that it wasn't just their training that was important. Social status at birth could prevent easy assimilation into genteel society and an 'unsuitable' marriage could compound this. As the professional standing of the surgeon-apothecary grew, so did the numbers in training and as we will see later in this chapter, the profession became overcrowded, causing a drop in the fees a doctor could charge. The Industrial Revolution, as well as creating new ways in which a man, woman, or child, could become sick, also changed the ways in which the medical profession was required to work. At the beginning of the eighteenth century around one in five of the population lived in an urban area, but by the middle of the nineteenth, more than fifty per cent were town dwellers. Those working in a country practice often had to travel long distances to attend their patients and transport was generally horseback, or simply on foot. Their motivation was increased by the possibility that by extending their territory they could gather in additional patients, even 'stealing' them from competitors and thus increase the value of their own list. Travel might also be increased if a practitioner developed a specialism for which he was well known, and was thus consulted, even by competitors, at a greater distance.

In *Making a Medical Living*, Anne Digby examined the diaries of William Goodwin of Earl Soham in Suffolk, who recorded his journeys for the years 1787 to 1789. His 'home territory' could be compared to a present day surgery 'catchment area', or the area within which most of the regular patients lived. Goodwin's territory was about ten miles by fifteen (around 150 square miles), but Digby calculates that there was a 'borderland', or larger area where the population might occasionally ask him for medical help. His diaries show that he travelled as far afield as Bungay, on the Norfolk border, and Southwold on the coast. This increases his total mileage to some thirty miles by thirty-five – a huge 1,000 square miles, and Digby was unable to identify any particular reason why Goodwin had been the surgeon of choice in those areas. It was likely that he had a good reputation but, if travelling on horseback, those distances equate to a journey of some four or five hours, and when roads were not made up or maintained, these were exhausting and potentially dangerous – accidents could be a frequent occurrence. Time spent recovering would mean greater opportunities for competitors to encroach.

The life of any ordinary practitioner was a difficult one and quite unlike the working life of the most eminent physicians to wealthy patients, who could relax in a carriage or, even if exertion was required, could at least expect to be well paid for his trouble. Cartoons of the period concentrate on these elite physicians who would treat their hypochondriac patients with unnecessary medicines and charge them exorbitant fees for the privilege. If looking closely at the regular GP, or surgeon-apothecary, of the time it is hard to reconcile the two.

Appointments under the Poor Law were very important as a source of income, not just to the newly qualified, but also as a regular source of supplementary income to the more established surgeon-apothecary. Before 1834, when the new Poor Law was introduced, there were around 15,000 parishes, each of whom could appoint a doctor to serve the population. Men could, therefore, represent more than one parish, and thereby increase their income. Some held appointments with as many as twelve different parishes, but the new Poor Law caused the gradual reduction of these parishes, as they were amalgamated in 600 unions, each with a number of medical districts. In 1844 the number of surgeons employed by the unions stood at 108, and there were significant inequalities of cover, which was addressed only gradually over the century.

Digby also looked at the different types of surgery available and the ways in which social standing was affected by the area within which a man found himself working. As previously mentioned, the surgery that relied on cash paying patients, perhaps sited in a large town or port, was the very bottom end of the medical market. Digby suggests that the slightly more fortunate practitioner would treat both the working-class and middle-class population in his area, supplementing his income with a Poor Law appointment. Above this, Digby places the 'suburban, middle-class practice with a range of appointments, or an unopposed (without competition, and therefore more valuable should the doctor seek to sell or take on an associate) country practice, preferably in good sporting country' (perhaps similar to that run by the Weekes family, see Chapter 9). The most prestigious general practice would be 'well established' and 'in a hospital town where there was hope of prestigious appointments', or 'fashionable' with wealthy patients, at the seaside or, like Jephson in Leamington Spa (see Chapter 7), at a popular place to take the waters.

In addition to those struggling to make a successful business based on a local population and Poor Law appointments, there were those who felt themselves sufficiently well connected, or well qualified, to anticipate a more prestigious appointment, as surgeon to one of the burgeoning number of county hospitals, such as Hereford, Exeter or Norwich. J.G. Crosse, a GP with a reputation in obstetrics, spent many years fostering the patronage of one Dr Rigby before being appointed Assistant Surgeon to the Norfolk and Norwich Hospital at the second time of trying. Even then, his private practice did not grow as quickly as he had hoped, but after three years he was promoted to Surgeon and had a successful career as a doctor specialising both in obstetrics and the treatment of the 'stone'. This system of patronage as a route to success was, as is usual in any career, a divisive one, and there was concern that skill had little to do with success in gaining a lucrative position at a hospital. It was one's connections that held the most weight, and if they involved family, so much the better because in some areas a post was held by generations of the same family. Elections required a significant amount of work on the part of the applicant for the position, and many continued their training whilst they waited, often as assistants in positions similar to that of the present day junior doctor, for a vacancy to become available and whilst they tried to build up a sufficiently lucrative private practice.

However, the 'assistant' became a vital member of the 'staff' in many a country medical practice, even in the earlier part of this period when apprentices were still available to do much of the 'donkey work' of the general practice. As Anne Digby states, they can easily be viewed as 'cheap labour', but for many, it was a wonderful way to gain additional experience and laid good foundations for those considering a career in their own general practice. Difficulties arose when the increasing number of hospitals, and therefore the additional supply of medical students, meant there were fewer openings for assistants, and they were less likely to become partners or take over their master's practice.

Building a successful general practice

For a 'general practice' to be successful, it was necessary to build up a significant source of income from private work, treating paying patients. This was often not just related to a medical man's standard of living, but also mattered as an indicator of social standing.

Other sources of income were available to the man determined to make his practice financially viable. These were the 'appointments' available in the local area and included that of medical officer to 'clubs' (for 'medical benefit'), factories, and mines. The most important were appointments under the Poor Laws.

Irvine Louden, in *Medical Care and the General Practitioner*, has undertaken some analysis of the impact of the 1834 Poor Law Act on the medical practice, and his work indicates that it was not only the Act itself that changed the environment for doctors and their patients, but the early nineteenth century hardening of attitudes towards the poor and the standard of proof they were required to meet when claiming relief. In a chilling analogy to the changes to the welfare system in the Britain of 2016, the 1834 Poor Law might refuse relief to a man recently operated on for an ulcerated tumour in his leg, the necessary walk to the hearing deciding his claim counting against him: if he could walk that far, he could work.

Irvine Louden queries Lindert and Williams's estimates of earnings in occupations over the period covered in this book, largely because they underestimate the earnings of a successful surgeon–apothecary GP in the late eighteenth century, setting the average salary at around £88. Their suggestion that earnings went up significantly in real terms is based on that figure when, Louden claims, earnings in excess of £300 were quite feasible. Therefore, it is more likely that average earnings in this branch of medicine remained in line with increased costs at best, and were more likely to have gone down. The eighteenth-century surgeon–apothecary was almost certainly better off than his general practitioner counterpart in the nineteenth century. Certainly, in *The Parent's Handbook*, published in 1842, the warning was given:

> *...there is no profession in which it is so difficult to make a beginning than that of medicine, and there is much truth in the saying that by the time when a physician earns his bread and cheese he has no longer the teeth to eat them with.*

Again, Louden suggests that this significant turnaround in fortunes, despite the speed with which medical care was advancing, was the 'excess of medical practitioners on market forces', and that 'excessive competition' affected what a man could earn even under Poor Law legislation.

Local county Register Offices hold Parish records of administration before 1834 so they are not easily searchable over a wide area. However, it seems clear from research undertaken by different researchers at different times that before 1834, the parishes offered a payment scheme that incentivised doctors to treat the poor with care. They could bill the parish for individual aspects of the care provided and in many cases, the fee would be comparable to that charged to a private patient.

Ordinary complaints, such as a cure for constipation, or a poultice for a boil, might be dealt with in the first instance by the local 'irregular practitioner', such as the untrained local 'nurse' or 'bone-setter', who may also have been responsible for the treatment of a patient's livestock. A professional doctor might be called in for the more complicated cases, and in some areas, where the setting of a broken bone might involve weeks out of work, the parish might be willing to provide the equivalent of 'sick pay' for the weeks of inactivity. In some areas, caution prevailed and to prevent weeks of payment to patients recovering after a botched job, the local doctor would be paid a part fee – the whole to be paid when treatment was successful. (This smacked of 'trade' however, and would be seen as a setback for the upwardly-mobile young doctor). A generous parish might pay for the alcohol necessary to dull the pain of an amputation, and then the wooden leg necessary to get a patient walking. Records, examined by E.G. Thomas, also show payments to the blind to learn the violin, and a pension to an elderly woman 'on account of her eyesight being bad which renders her incapable of doing anything for a livelihood'. (E.G. Thomas *The Old Poor Law and Medicine* 1980.)

The parish authorities seem, from a number of examples to have been generous in their payments. In one parish, in addition to the fee to the midwife, the parish also paid for candles, beer, and a grocer's bill.

There was little oversight of the care provided, but if the parish were a small one and a doctor's reputation hard won, there was little reason to scrimp, even though the treatment of wealthier patients may have been undertaken more carefully, with an eye to increasing social stature.

To illustrate his point, Louden examined county records in Bedfordshire and Wiltshire and discovered significant payments made to a Dr McGrath, who was surgeon to seven Bedfordshire parishes with a total population of around 3,500, only ten per cent of whom were eligible for poor relief. In 1811 he received over £100 for his work – a significant sum equating to more than £5,000 today. At this time, payment was by a combination of salary and by item of treatment, but men like McGrath were to gradually see that shift further towards salary only. Parish salaries were around £10–15 per annum, so to have responsibility for more parishes meant the sums could add up, and with additional payments for setting broken bones, for example, a parish could pay as much as £100 per annum. However, in changing times, this benevolent attitude was not to last. Despite much blame being attached to the Poor Law of 1834, it seems that was but a crystallisation of a change in attitudes towards the poor that began in the second decade of the century. Despite, or perhaps because of, the rising numbers of medical students qualifying, it was possible for parishes to put the position of surgeon out to tender and take the lowest bidder, often over the much more experienced local man. The standard of care available to the poor was reduced along with the salaries, and the belief that the poor 'got what they deserved' became more widespread.

The Poor Law Act of 1834 is notorious for the brutal attitude it took towards poverty and the poor, many of whom, it felt, had been encouraged into idleness by the previous administration of relief by the parishes. It surely can't be a coincidence that at the same time as this legislation was being drafted, another Act – the Anatomy Act of 1832 – declared that even in death the earthly body of a pauper was at the mercy of the state and could be dissected and dismembered in the name of science (see Chapter 3).

The Poor Law has, down the decades since its passing, been examined in detail; its intentions have been analysed and the results graphically described and roundly condemned. Comparisons with the twenty-first-century reforms to the welfare system are chilling in their similarities; both attempt to reduce the escalating costs of caring for those unable to work, claiming that new restrictions affect only the able-bodied who could find work if they were minded to. Relief available after 1834 was not to amount to more than the average pay offered in the most menial of labouring jobs and at all stages of the process, the possibility of an abuse of the system (rather than a genuine assessment of need) was to be paramount. Life for the able-bodied poor was not to be one of any comfort – outdoor relief was practically abolished, so the workhouse gradually became the only, dreaded, option for the poorest. The workhouse infirmary became a repository for the sick poor who could no longer rely on a doctor visiting them at home, and that ugly distinction between 'deserving' and 'undeserving' poor became the source of much unfairness and discrimination. As Irvine Louden states:

The pretence that a clear distinction could be made between the undeserving pauper and the deserving poor did more than anything else to limit and degrade the new poor law medical service. The sick poor were inevitably, if unintentionally, subjected to a harshness for which no excuse can be found, and which persisted into the twentieth century.

The sick poor came to be viewed as somehow ill through their own fault – this coming at a time of great change in the structure of society during the industrial revolution when men found myriad new ways to create opportunities for accidents and increased vulnerability to disease.

The replacement of around 10,000 parishes with 2,500 'Unions' (of parishes) resulted in a significant reduction in the number of medical officers employed. Irvine Louden:

'The reduction of Poor Law medical posts after 1834 was from sixteen to three in Lincoln, from sixteen to seven in Bridgwater, from sixteen to three in Aylesbury…from ten to two in Shipston, and from twelve to six in Newbury.'

These reductions allowed unions to drastically reduce the costs of providing medical care to the sick poor. Louden again:

In 1844 the number of available posts as surgeon to a union in England was about 2,400. The average salary was £69 per annum. When this is compared to the salaries paid to parish surgeons at the end of the eighteenth century it can be seen at once that payment per unit of population was much lower…

He goes on to point out that the union man had four or five times as many patients under his care than the old parish surgeon had for the same money. These increased workloads and reduction in salary still did not deter men from applying for vacant positions, and it was still seen as an important stepping-stone in the career of a young man keen to build up a successful private practice. Many held their positions for only as long as it took to build up a sufficient base of fee-paying patients or more attractive appointments.

The new Poor Law required doctors to provide dressings and drugs within the salary they were paid so it was, therefore, likely that some treatments might have been withheld from the poorest. Travel expenses could not be claimed separately so many union doctors never travelled to the further reaches of their parish and patients felt less inclined to call in a stranger in any event. Medical treatment would inevitably suffer.

Many of the doctors employed in the role of surgeon to the parish were well-meaning souls who wanted to treat all their patients with equal care; but the union system, which might reduce the payment per patient to as little as 7d per case after expenses made such benevolence impossible. Local Boards were not even responsible for assessing the number of surgeons necessary to adequately cover their populations – that decision was taken higher up; in London, despite there being a ready pool of applicants willing to take on the job, more experienced men were undercut and priced out of the market.

Irvine Louden uses the town of Huddersfield as an example of the total indifference to, and scorn felt for, both patients and surgeons by a Board of Governors keen to squeeze every penny of value from their appointees. In 1843, a Mr Tatham was medical officer to the northern division of the Huddersfield Union. The salary was £40 per annum and Tatham was required to pay for any medicines he prescribed. In his first year, he made more than 1,600 journeys and paid for drugs to a total value of £37 18s 7d. Thus his profit was around £2 per annum. When he requested a pay rise he was refused the requested, and reasonable, sum of £70, being allowed just £50, which rose gradually to £80. Tatham was not to enjoy the benefits of any increase, however. The building of a fever hospital (the Huddersfield area experienced a high number of cases of typhus at the time) and Tatham's responsibility for admissions to it (running at an average of twenty-seven per week) left him in the red. He was in effect subsidising the union, who, when Tatham asked for an additional salary to cover the costs, turned him down flat. He sued the Board, but lost on a technicality, frustrating both judge and jury who considered the Board's treatment of their medical man to be totally wrong.

Apart from the necessity to gain experience, and the willingness of the newly qualified to take on these roles, what might possess a man to accept the fact that he must be overworked, underpaid, and frustrated in any attempt he might make to improve the lot of the poor? There was the possibility that the position might lead to better connections, and a more respected position in society and one's work ethic could not be queried. In other areas, a man might take on the job to ensure he was free from competition from other general practitioners in his areas, exclusivity being such a valuable commodity in a practice – he would do it simply to make sure no one else could. Some very benevolent men became Union doctors just because they loved the job, even where it did not pay, but they would almost certainly have had another source of income.

Overall, the system of medical provision to the poor after the Act of 1834 was a failure and a cruel one. At a time when, by all accounts, there were more than enough general practitioners being trained, the union system was allowed to remain grossly understaffed.

Making a living in medicine

The income of the Weekes family (Chapter 9) has been examined in some detail by John M.T. Ford, but as no account books or day books from the firm have survived, their total income has had to remain vague. There is little doubt that the family was comfortably off, but Richard Weekes, and later his sons, worked very hard for whatever they did earn. The sons were educated in the best schools possible and their careers in medicine supported by their father's earnings. Hampton Weekes regularly sent home items from London that were costly and unavailable in Sussex, and there were trips to theatres, and stays in fashionable towns and cities. With little reliance on parish work (a total of around £60 per annum is suggested from the parish accounts), the private patients in the area seem likely to have ensured that the Weekes' family income was in excess of the average at the time (calculated to be around £260 pa). When he died, Richard Weekes Snr was able to leave land to both his sons and substantial annuities in trust for his unmarried daughter. By the late Victorian period, the Weekes' family medical dynasty had accumulated three large houses, smaller tenanted properties, and wealthy connections by marriage.

Salaries

Becoming a doctor did not guarantee a lucrative career. Matthew Flinders (1750–1802), of Donington in Lincolnshire, was the grandson of a farmer and son of a surgeon. In 1770 he took over his father's practice and kept detailed financial records. In his first year, he earned just £72, a figure which rose to £582 by the end of the eighteenth century. Some successful physicians and surgeons earned over £1,000, although apothecaries earned less and in the countryside such incomes were rarer, and the work desperately hard, as a doctor may have many miles to cover on horseback or on foot. Much of the work undertaken by junior doctors, on the wards of a hospital or infirmary was unpaid and even into the twentieth century, doctors working in poorer areas, or taking up a residency in a hospital, would earn much less than Matthew Flinders.

Research has shown that doctors in the nineteenth century were on the whole better off than doctors in the twenty-first century. The same study suggests that the fortunes of individual doctors varied wildly. For example, Arthur Hill Hassall, physician and microscopist left just £55 at his death, whilst Sir William Jenner, physician, left £385,083. The two men were direct contemporaries, both living almost the length of the nineteenth century.

Chapter 5

What could the surgeon-apothecary treat? Eighteenth and nineteenth century medical treatments

From the relative comfort of the twenty-first century and the medical advances we enjoy now, it is both horrific and fascinating to learn about the conditions, concerns and 'cures' that were part of life (and death) for our forebears.

Details are often lacking in the general histories of medicine, and the biographies of medical men, but in this chapter it has been possible to look at the most common illnesses recorded and the possible treatments offered, owing, in part, to the detailed studies made by Irvine Louden in *Medical Care and the General Practitioner 1750-1850*, and by the family of Robert Storrs, surgeon apothecary of Doncaster (see chapter 7), in *Humane and Heroic*, by John Tooth. Louden has gathered morbidity statistics from the period, and Tooth has made use of Storrs's fulsome records and diaries held at the Wellcome Library.

There are also certain illnesses and diseases that were prevalent in the eighteenth and nineteenth century, but which we rarely see today. Some have different names, and many are now deemed to be minor inconveniences rather than life threatening conditions.

Real progress was not made in the treatment of some of these conditions until the development of antibiotics in the 1920s, and some were still causing death and lifelong health problems well into the twentieth century.

So what could the eighteenth and early nineteenth century medic hope to 'cure'? In *Medical Care and the General Practitioner*, Irvine Louden states that the only specific treatments that we would consider useful in the twenty-first century are quinine (effective in treating malaria), digitalis (used to treat dropsy, possibly as a result of heart failure), fresh fruit and vegetable (for scurvy and their obvious health benefits) and opium (as pain relief, as a sedative, or even as a stimulant). In addition, the smallpox vaccine developed in this period saved millions of lives.

So when the list of treatments regularly offered by doctors is examined, there was, at best, a vast quantity of generally harmless but unnecessary (and often ghastly) medicines consumed, and at worst, a number of potentially deadly poisons taken.

For example, The Old Operating Theatre Museum offers an eighteenth-century recipe for the treatment of a 'venereal disease':

Snail Water

Take Garden-Snails cleansed and bruised 6 gallons,

Earthworms washed and bruised 3 gallons,

Of common Wormwood, Ground-Ivy, and Carduus [Aster], each one Pound,

Penniroyal, Juniper-berries, Fennelseeds, Aniseeds, each half a pound,

Cloves and Cubebs [a pepper] bruised, each 3 ounces,

Spirit of Wine and Spring-water, of each 8 Gallons,

Digest them together for the space of 24 Hours,

And then draw it off in a common Alembick [a still]

Further examples are given in Appendix 1.

There are many cartoons and prints drawn and painted in the eighteenth and nineteenth centuries suggesting that in many cases practitioners were well aware of the limitations of the remedies they prescribed, often at significant cost to the patient. Richard Smith, chief surgeon at the Bristol Royal Infirmary from 1835 to 1843 was, as a surgeon rather than a physician, scathing:

> ...*even the London and Edinburgh pharmacopoeias were loaded with a miserable farrago of useless trash ... Three-fourths of the medicines purchased of the Druggist were mere adulterations ... opium, antimony, mercury and many others when needful, of course, employed ... but the great bulk of bottles were mere placebos...*
>
> (from Louden p 64)

When the dispensing of medicines formed the larger part of a medical man's income, it is possible some were exploiting the health anxieties of their patients, particularly if they were physician to a wealthy family or individual. Only a minority of doctors charged for the medicines alone – most would add a call out fee and additional charges should procedures such as bleeding, or a clyster (an enema), be required. But with a population prone to hypochondria, and with death ever present in their lives, it is hardly surprising if, when a livelihood depended on it, a doctor prescribed a potion or lotion not yet proved to be efficacious. Besides, as in the twenty first century, the 'placebo' effect often produced seemingly good results.

Thomas Marryat, eighteenth-century surgeon, and writer, in his book *Therapeutics; or, the Art of healing* first published in 1813 says some interesting things about the role of the physician in the art of blending ingredients to good effect, but has to admit that at times, things work without explanation:

> *With respect to the mode of operations of medicines it must be confessed we are somewhat in the dark; the human body is too complicated a machine to be amenable to those laws which solids and fluids out of it may be subject to. Those who tread the high priori* [self-evident without the need for reasoning] *road are mighty apt to grow giddy and stumble. Nature is very often exceedingly unmannerly to theories... Would it not be more ingenious to acknowledge that medicines do generally produce effects, though we cannot satisfactorily account for the manner in which they act? ... A man much conversant in the practice of physic might recite many narratives of the operations of drugs which would hazard his credit... Nevertheless their power ... is by no means inconsiderable and it seems as novel for physicians to inveigh against the use of drugs, as for a man of learning to decry erudition... When a person is ill. He naturally and justly looks for the restoration of his health from a physician, and the number of those who are disappointed in comparatively exceedingly small.*

Helpless as they were in the face of infections, fevers and countless other debilitating diseases, doctors resorted to preparations that they knew offered, at the very least, comfort to the concerned patient. For many, the mere presence of the doctor by the sickbed produced restorative effects and much of their work was simply to reassure.

Surgery

> *Of the agony it occasioned I will say nothing. Suffering so great as I underwent cannot be expressed in words, and thus fortunately cannot be recorded. The particular pangs are no forgotten; but the black whirlwind*

of emotion, the horror of great darkness, and the sense of desertion by God and man, bordering close upon despair, which swept through my mind and overwhelmed my heart, I can never forget, however gladly I would do so.,

(from a letter from an 'old patient' to
J.Y. Simpson quoted in Louden p 73)

A reader of popular medical history is used to hearing the horror stories of operations undertaken at the famous hospital medical schools. The vision of a poor patient held down on the operating table, un-anaesthetised, cut and sewn up as quickly as possible to avoid blood loss and shock is gruesome in the extreme. Descriptions of Samuel Pepys's operation for the 'stone' or Fanny Burney's mastectomy are repeated regularly as an indication of the horrors of medicine before the introduction of more modern methods; however, for the surgeon–apothecary of the small community or provincial hospital, such serious operations were a rare occurrence. It was more likely that our medical man would be treating a leg ulcer or an injury following an accident. Few patients would need more than rest and medicinal preparations to support recovery. Irvine Louden examines the caseload of John Wright, surgeon to the Nottingham General Hospital. Of 152 cases admitted between 1795 and 1797, only four needed a major operation, including a 35-year-old male for the removal of an injured testicle and a 37-year-old woman who had her leg amputated. Forty-four patients were treated for leg ulcers, forty-eight for accidents and orthopaedic conditions and thirty-eight with a variety of medical disorders, such as venereal disease and cancers.

William Pulsford, from Wells in Somerset, worked in partnership with his uncle Benjamin Pulsford in the 1750-60s. One ledger has survived from their practice and analysis of its contents indicates that of 334 new cases, twenty-seven per cent were as a result of accidents, including fractures, dislocations, burns, and cuts and bruises caused largely by falls from, or kicks by, horses. Falls, fights and guns were also responsible, but only two cases needed a major operation.

The seemingly disproportionate number of patients suffering from leg ulcers has been studied in detail by Louden, and he contends that although not specified, these ulcers were the result of quite different conditions to those experienced, mainly by the elderly population, today. Tuberculosis, syphilis and a dietary deficiency could affect a far younger group of patients and they were often very difficult to cure.

Pulsford's ledger also offers a picture of his daily life, much of which seems to be taken up with visits to these surgical patients, some of whom seem unable to deal with even the most minor strain or pain without resort to Pulsford's services; so much the better for his annual income.

Other common surgical cases included tooth extraction, the draining of boils and abscesses, and the dressing of wounds, as well as venesection, or bloodletting. This minor surgery could be effective, and evidence suggests it was, in the late eighteenth century at least, lucrative.

London surgeons were known to charge hundreds of pounds for an operation, but these were not to treat conditions most often seen by the local general practitioner. His surgical work was regular and payment was often for small amounts. As seen in Chapter 4, the fees, if not the treatment, were broadly the same for both rich and poor patient, and across the country.

For example, William Pulsford of Wells charged one and a half guineas to treat a child who had dislocated their wrist falling from a tree and five guineas for a gunshot wound to the hand. Opening an abscess could cost anything from five shillings to one and a half guineas, and the on-going treatment for an ulcerated leg cost fourteen guineas over two-and-a-half years. Parish work was charged out at the same rate as private work and in 1757, it made Pulsford more than twenty guineas. As mentioned in Chapter 4, a GP's income was dependent on fees from a number of different sources, and William Pulsford was practising at a time when the old Poor Law administration was still relatively generous. As competition grew, fees could not go up in line with increased costs, so it is difficult to compare the fees of 1757 with those of later periods. However, five shillings paid in 1757 would be worth approximately £20 in 2015 and might be two days wages for a skilled artisan of the time. (National Archives Currency Converter.)

The Man-Midwife

The image of an eighteenth or nineteenth century midwife (apart from that of the notoriously dissolute and incompetent Sarah Gamp in *Martin Chuzzlewit* by Charles Dickens) is frequently that of a stern woman, marshalling a young assistant and refusing entry to the woman's bedroom to anyone unnecessary to the birth – including (and most importantly) any men of the house. Very often, for the poorest, a local woman with some experience of childbirth would be the best help they could afford. However, by the end of the eighteenth century, local GPs or surgeons had taken on the role, at least in market towns and more rural areas. There may still have been a fair ratio of midwives to doctors, but by the turn of the century, it was rare to find a surgeon-apothecary who was not also a man-midwife.

A man-midwife, particularly in fashionable circles, was also known as an *accoucheur* from the French 'to go to bed' or 'to be delivered'. During the eighteenth century, the rise of obstetrics as a suitable subject for study and the role of midwife proper for a man was dramatic. The reason for the rise is open to debate, but could include men's increasing confidence with surgical techniques, the development and improvement of the forceps as a tool to aid a natural birth, and market forces – in the sense that, in an increasingly competitive market, it was a new discipline to seek expertise in and an area within which, if successful, a new and fruitful source of patients would result.

Many people felt strongly that the place by the side of a woman during childbirth should be taken by a woman. There was not just anger from midwives, who saw their position taken away. Many doctors felt that attendance at a long, and probably natural, labour was a waste of valuable time, which a doctor could better spend on other patients who needed him for a genuine medical reason. Others felt there was something 'unmanly' about a doctor who wanted to take on this role. Some thought there were what we would now refer to as gender politics involved, in that as a man had been the primary cause of the discomfort, and any possible complications, he could not justify further intervention. Strangely, the objections seem only rarely to be a result of delicacy. Although, as we shall see, childbirth was changed to ensure the male midwife was not accused of, or tempted into, impropriety, there was an acknowledgement that he would have access to a woman's body in order to diagnose other complaints; as long as the role of medic and patient were strictly adhered to, there should be no concerns.

A little snippet from the *Caledonian Mercury* of 19 July 1776 offers this interesting view. Under the heading 'The Man-Midwife an ANECDOTE':

A Lady who had two children, at her third lying-in, was persuaded to change her midwife for a man-midwife; accordingly the great Dr __ __ was sent for; when he had got almost to the chamber door, he was stopped by her Ladyship's maid who begged to know of him whether he was a married man or not; to which he replied, that indeed he was not married, but he kept a lady. The maid acquainted her mistress therewith, who made answer, 'That it was just the same as if he was married if he kept a lady' and desired the Doctor to be shewn in...

This is an interesting indicator of a rather confused attitude to male morals in the second half of the eighteenth century. Presumably, a single man of little experience would not be so welcome.

In another case, a woman's refusal to admit a man-midwife may have cost her her life. Her (female) midwife was taken before the King's Bench in 1789, 'for using instruments in the delivery of a woman by which she died'. However, all agreed that the birth had been a difficult case, and as the patient had refused to admit a man who may have been able to help, no blame could be attached to the midwife, and she was found not guilty. (*Norfolk Chronicle* 11 July 1789.)

The significant rise in importance of the man-midwife is all the more remarkable for the lack of support offered by the Colleges and corporations for those taking up obstetrics. Scotland accepted the importance of the subject to their students and offered courses in obstetrics long before it was accepted south of the border, where arguments about who was responsible for training also held up education and research. The physicians at the Royal College believed the messy business to be the province of the surgeon, although they would deign to be involved if there were problems during the pregnancy or after the birth.

The surgeons were not keen to take on the role either. The Company of Surgeons, later the Royal College of Surgeons, wanted to restrict their members to undertaking 'pure' surgery, but in reality neither branch of the profession considered it a 'manly' role and it was therefore work only fit for the lower ranks. This attitude continued into the nineteenth century and eventually, the role became one central to the general practice.

There has been a considerable amount of historical debate about how the man-midwife so effectively usurped the role of the woman assistant during childbirth. There is no ready answer, and as Lisa Forman Cody says in *Birthing the Nation: Sex, Science, and the Conception of Eighteenth-Century Britain* the two dominant historical arguments are poles apart:

> *From the time man-midwives began giving obstetric lectures in the eighteenth century, proponents trumpeted the triumphs of the profession; forceps, fillets, education, masculine ingenuity, and emotional detachment. Naturally, sensible fathers to be and their pregnant wives chose obstetricians. From the 1960s onward, many women's historians echoed Elizabeth Nihall's 1760 argument. Obstetricians denigrated midwives, magnetically described their own charms, unnecessarily wielded instruments, cruelly thrust them into women, and often killed mothers and infants.*

Cody labels these versions 'medical glory versus gory misogyny', and neither is a historically accurate explanation. It would be remarkable, Cory asserts, if women continued to allow a male midwife near her if he was known to hack up other women and their babies. Equally, with all we know of the modesty surrounding sex at the time, there must have been more than medical bravura about a man to enable him to convince a woman that she can trust him at such an important time?

It was, of course, easier for the female midwife to examine a woman fully. Some allowed the woman to choose the birthing position she found most comfortable, and the birthing stool was a common item used, offering a comfortable position and allowing gravity to assist in the delivery. As the male midwife became more common, the generally accepted position for delivery was changed to one that many would find far less comfortable. The woman had to lie on her side, with her face away from the doctor in attendance. Doctors were also more reluctant to undertake abdominal examinations in case it led to accusations of impropriety, an issue that could lead to life-threatening misdiagnosis.

A man must also develop a charming bedside manner to ensure the patient's confidence, and many did this by ordering about the female nurse (who might once have been the midwife) or lady's maid. Sarah Stone wrote angrily of a newly qualified surgeon-apothecary that he 'puts on a finished assurance that their knowledge exceeds any woman's'.

Midwives of the early eighteenth century sensed that they might be partly responsible for the 'fashion' for having a man at the birth. Lack of confidence in difficult cases often led a midwife to call in a doctor before it was necessary, and thus pass any credit for her own skill to the man-midwife. Sarah Stone also considered that forceps – used solely by the man-midwife, were used far too frequently, a fact endorsed, ironically, in the lectures given by two of the leading obstetricians of the period, Smellie and Hunter, who tried to discourage their students from unnecessary interventions.

It seems likely that the male midwife was better able to listen to a woman's general concerns about the medical aspects of childbirth, and able to calm them, seeming to be more of a friend than a nurse. Women were, and still are, influenced by their friend's experience of childbirth, and once a man–midwife had safely delivered a number of babies in his area, he was most likely the subject of conversations at female gatherings. As Cody says 'Man-midwives, as it turns out did rather well by word of mouth and public recommendations'.

But the man-midwife was not always the triumphant master of his female counterpart. For many doctors, the role was an unpleasant chore; something that had to be taken on if the practice was to be profitable.

'The man-midwife … cannot be compensated at all by the mere lying-in fee, unless it leads to other business. I know of no surgeon who would not willingly have given up attending midwifery cases provided he could retain the family in other respects…' (Richard Smith of Bristol quoted in Louden.)

Certainly, in many country areas, the doctor had to attend when called, regardless of whether his skills were required or not. Matthew Flinders of Lincolnshire notes in his diary that he had spent forty hours without sleep, attending two normal births. This was at a fee between just 10s 6d and a guinea per case.

Looking at the Weekes family letters (see Chapter 9) it was clear that they charged a higher fee to wealthier patients – 15s for a parish baby and five guineas for delivery to a wealthier family, although the higher fee would doubtless include considerably more ante-natal and post-natal care and attendance at false alarms could not be charged as extra.

Other records, such as those of Danvers Ward of Bristol, indicate that a man may work in the field simply for the love of it. Ward was clearly keen on the obstetric arm of his practice, the records available showing that over a third of his cases were obstetric and in one year he delivered 121 women, at a fee of between half a guinea and three guineas, and despite the lengthy period usually necessary to deliver a baby and the speedy nature of many of his other non-obstetric cases – dental extractions and abscesses for example – his average fee in both cases was around 14s 6d. He, and other doctors, also delivered babies free of charge to the poorest families, indicating a genuine love for childbirth.

In the nineteenth century, the role of the GP in obstetric cases grew until it became an exhausting but vital source of work in a successful practice.

Chapter 6

Quack Quack – the medical profession and a battle for the pennies of the poor patent medicines

As to Squire Western, he was seldom out of the sick-room, unless when he was engaged either in the field or over his bottle. Nay, he would sometimes retire hither to take his beer, and it was not without difficulty that he was prevented from forcing Jones to take his beer too: for no quack ever held his nostrum to be a more general panacea than he did this; which, he said, had more virtue in it than was in all the physic in an apothecary's shop.

(Tom Jones, Henry Fielding)

There is ground enough in this huge town for the detector of quackery to exercise his art, nobody will venture to deny; and there can be no fear of any dearth of game; only let him beware that he does not, like the London sportsmen, pour his random shot on unlawful game. Though Mr Corry is a good marksman in general, this caution may be great service to him; since he is apt sometimes to be careless in taking aim. To be serious, there are names in this little book, which we should never have expected to see in such company, unless it were by way of contrast to the rest; which is not the case...

The second quote at the start of this chapter neatly sums up the difficulties facing those determined to expose 'quackery' and quack doctors in the late eighteenth and throughout the nineteenth century. John Corry was the author of *The detector of quackery*, published in 1802 and determined to expose fraud, not just in the medical profession, but across a wide range of the arts and science. An Irish-born writer and journalist, Corry wrote the *'detector'* as a 'well-intended satire [to] rouse the public to just indignation against the quacks and their abettors'. He said that 'Quack doctors', some of whom he mentions by name, 'practise their fraudulent arts with most success in a wealthy commercial country like England, especially in the busy populous and luxurious capital, where the multitude have neither leisure or inclination to detect imposture'.

Corry was determined, by such satirical exposure, to alert the population to the dangers inherent in a number of medicines, available directly from a sales person or via newspaper advertisements, and given credence or support by legal patent. The medical profession was, in this period, still riven by disagreement as to its structure and the relative value of titles given to medical men within it. Degrees in medicine could be 'bought' from colleges only interested in the payment of fees and Corry considered that many were being duped into using these men instead of the 'regular' trained and experienced doctor, whether physician, surgeon or apothecary.

As the decades passed he was joined by other zealous voices calling for the outlawing of those who traded in and benefitted financially from, the misery and ill health of others, knowing how little their treatments might help. Little did he know when he wrote his pamphlets and pursued his campaign, that the medicines he so despised would still be sold and relied upon, particularly by the poor and the working class, well into the twentieth century.

Some medicines, and those who sold them, were obviously fraudulent; at best useless and at worst positively dangerous. Others were much harder to define or expose. If it was not possible to explain clearly the meaning of 'quack', how could it be eradicated? This chapter looks at some of the men who tried to reduce the public's reliance on proprietary or patent medicines and ensure that that the medical profession was properly regulated to protect the public from those unqualified to provide treatment.

Attacks upon the community of 'irregular' practitioners – those midwives, chemists nurses and 'horse-doctors' who had practised healing in their local areas for many years – began in earnest at the end of the eighteenth century, and continued well into the nineteenth. It has to be remembered that when the attack was on traditional providers of medical care, rancour was often stirred up by the medical profession itself, under threat from above by increased political pressure to reorganise, reform and regulate, and from below by the many they perceived to be unqualified and untrained. Other chapters have highlighted how far the medical profession was from any unified or regulated structure in this period. At the top of the profession there were the 'elite' practitioners, closely guarding their privilege, and the fortunes that privilege brought with it. In the middle were the 'regulars' – those working in small towns and villages, trained as surgeons or apothecaries – who performed the function of general practitioner to the population of the areas they served, often at the expense of their own health and for only a modest, if not lowly, remuneration. At the bottom were the 'irregulars' and these were the ones most easily labelled as 'quacks' by those higher up the structure of the medical profession.

For example, in the John Johnson Collection, held at the Bodleian Library, is an advert placed around 1780, by 'J. Dalton, chemist and druggist, (from London,) King-Street, Richmond, Surrey'. Wearing his London credentials proudly, he wishes to inform 'the nobility, gentry, and public', 'that he prepares and sells every article in the medical line, on the same terms as in London'. Typically, Mr Galton then proceeds to recommend his 'horse medicines, which are kept ready prepared, agreeable to the Recipes of the most eminent Farriers…'

His products include 'diuretic or urine balls', 'purging balls with rhubarb' and 'pectoral balls for coughs, or asthmatic and thick-winded horses'.

These were over-the-counter remedies that required no prescription from any doctor, however well qualified, and it was therefore not surprising that many who had undertaken a lengthy period as apprentice felt threatened in what was an already over-crowded market.

Irvine Louden points out the challenges the qualified doctor faced at this time. Medical schools first established in Scotland and then in the capital and larger cities across Britain, oversupplied what could be called the 'medical market' with doctors qualifying in their expensive establishments. Many blamed the introduction of the Apothecaries Act of 1815 for making the medical profession too popular, and although that was not the sole reason, there was a significant increase in the number of young men attending the various schools in the first decades of the nineteenth century. There was little incentive to limit or regulate the numbers; the schools were in competition with one another and with the glut of qualified men, many returning home from serving as medical officers in the army or navy, came pressure on the charges they could make to their patients. It became a 'patient's market', and there were dedicated doctors worn out by the constant need to secure a viable list of the sick – who were also often poor.

As Louden says, it is very difficult to say who exactly the true 'quacks' were. In his exhaustive research, he could not identify them from membership lists as they were not in the habit of forming associations, or of writing diaries or memoirs, as many doctors did, and their accounts are non-existent. Louden has to rely on the wonderful collection of pamphlets held in the Bodleian Library in Oxford. He notes particularly the success of 'Dr' Solomon of Liverpool who made his fortune making and selling the 'Cordial Balm of Gilead', of which Louden says: 'If you were ill the balm cured you; if down in the dumps it cheered you up.' His genius was in advertising and said he could spend £100 on adverts to bring in £2,000 of profit. But he was not alone.

Research using the John Johnson Collection at the Bodleian offers a fascinating insight into the medical treatments endured during the eighteenth and nineteenth centuries. It is no use us being smug, in the heady days of the twenty-first century, when we still insist on a prescription for antibiotics to treat a virus, or take up ten minutes of our GP's time because our eating habits have caused symptoms we could easily have avoided by a change in diet or the use of an over the counter laxative, made from the same ingredients our nineteenth century ancestors would have been familiar with.

So when we read contemporaneous accounts of the horrors of the 'quack', it is useful to understand first whom the author of the account is. The doctors were not unbiased observers of this additional, unwanted, layer of competition.

The Lancet, under the control of Thomas Wakley, was a journal at the forefront of the campaign against the continued success of the 'irregular' in the 1820s. Wakley was a surgeon and acted as coroner in a number of cases where death appeared to have been directly caused by an over the counter, proprietary medicine. These cases infuriated him into print, where he highlighted the tragedies caused by, in his words, a 'satanic system of quackery'. In many ways, he was right to focus on the 'sharp' end of the market, where manufacturers and purveyors of patent medicines were well aware that they were offering false hopes and taking money by deception.

Many of the traditional 'irregulars' genuinely believed they could help and were horrified if it seemed they were the cause of a tragedy.

One such irregular was a Mr Lowe, who, in 1846, was called to give evidence to an inquest into the death of Martha Grogan, aged 3. Martha was the daughter of a greengrocer, and it was alleged by her parents that she had died as a result of the effects of pills administered by Mr Lowe, a retired officer of the East India Company. The inquest was first adjourned to call Mr Lowe, who, the reports say 'was in his 94th year'. He was not well enough to attend, and was represented by his son, who said 'his father was the oldest inhabitant in the parish' who had lived in the same street for about 'half a century'. Throughout the whole period, he had

> ...*been in the constant habit of administering medical aid to the poor, gratis', that is, free of any charge. Mr Lowe's son said his father was well aware of the nature of the pills, and that they were not made by him, but by 'an eminent medical practitioner' and 'procured from the Apothecaries Hall'.*

Martha's mother was convinced the child was killed by the pills, despite having rushed Martha to King's College Hospital, where a Dr Farrar diagnosed the primary problem as a whooping cough, from which many children died. Farrar prescribed port and beef tea, which apparently made the child better, but only for a brief period. After her death, the parents continued to maintain that the pills prescribed by Mr Lowe had caused mercury poisoning and that that had been the cause of death.

Dr Farrar, when further questioned, maintained that despite a significant 'necrosis' around the jaw, this was better ascribed to the 'unhealthy districts' within which the Grogans lived, and the 'bad food' that Martha had been fed. He considered death to be by natural causes, despite an analysis of the pills showing that they were almost entirely hemlock and were highly poisonous.

The jury agreed with Dr Farrar, but added: 'We strongly reprobate the practice of Mr Lowe in administering medicines which were proved to be of an injurious character and the more so he being totally ignorant of medical practice.'

This was a case in which there was no satisfaction for anyone concerned. Lowe was chastised for his attempts at helping the poor of his parish, with no benefit to himself, and Martha and her parents were no nearer to having a conclusive diagnosis of the cause of her death.

Many of those who peddled the 'nostrums' were more businessman, or occasionally, woman, than doctor. It was their sales technique and their sheer bravura in making excessive claims about the effectiveness of their potions that distinguished them from the country herbalist or horse doctor. Wakley, in *The Lancet*, published the ingredients of many of the most popular brands. For example, 'Spilsbury's Antiscorbutic Drops', advertised widely as a treatment for scrofula, as a disease (associated with tuberculosis) of the lymph nodes, was exposed as made up almost entirely of antimony, a substance generally used as a purgative. 'Daffy's Elixir', marketed as a curative for flatulence and colic, might have the same effect, composed as it was of Senna leaves.

Dr James Parkinson (See Chapter 7) said of 'quacks' in his book *The Villager's Friend and Physician*:

> *Be assured, that for this disease* [breast cancer] *there is no remedy known. Medicines, which have been reported to have been used with success by quacks and others, have had the fairest trial by surgeons of the first abilities, but have been found unsuccessful. Notwithstanding this, cruel, daring and I may, with the strictest propriety, say, murderous quacks, are hourly pretending to cure this disease. I speak of the in*

> *language thus strong, because the mischief they occasion is not merely*
> *by employing improper means, but by deluding their unhappy patients*
> *into so firm a reliance on their nostrums, that they are induced to put*
> *aside all ideas of the removal of the diseased part, and to allow it, whilst*
> *deceived into a daily expectation of its cure, to degenerate into that*
> *dreadful state, which art possesses no power to alter...*

Wakley, in true tabloid style, went into battle with those supplying the useless and potentially dangerous remedies. He called to those living in even the smallest towns to expose local quacks in an attempt to put them out of business. Roy Porter in *Health for Sale* details the case of Dr Reynolds Fowler of Wiltshire, who sold his treatment for worms via newspaper adverts and stalls in local markets, where the local, seemingly worm-ridden, populous queued to take advantage of whatever properties Dr Reynolds Fowler's concoction claimed. It is to be hoped it was not in any way similar to Ching's Patent Worm Lozenges, as described by Caroline Rance on The QuackDoctor.com. Rance details how, according to the Hull Packet of 1 November 1803, a 3-year-old boy called Thomas Clayton was given Ching's lozenges by his parents, who repeated the dose three days later, only to see their son deteriorate in the most horrible way very soon afterwards:

> *...the mouth ulcerated, the Teeth dropped out, the Hands contracted,*
> *and a complaint was made, of a pricking Pain in them and the Feet,*
> *the Body became flushed and spotted, and at last Black Convulsions*
> *succeeded, attended with a slight delirium; and a mortification destroyed*
> *the face, which proceeding to the Brain, put a period (after indescribable*
> *torments) to the life of the little sufferer, on Sunday...Twenty-Eight*
> *Days after he had taken the Poisonous lozenges.*

The lozenges were sold by travelling agents, who were, Rance says 'under strict instruction' to reassure those buying them that they contained 'not a single particle of mercury'. However, the symptoms experienced by poor Thomas included classic indicators of mercury poisoning and the coroner came to the conclusion that the boy had indeed been 'Poisoned by Ching's Worm Lozenges'.

The boy's father spent many subsequent years campaigning to expose Ching's lozenges for the poison they were and wrote a pamphlet in 1805, offering a number of suggestions for the eradication of quackery, not least by reducing the government's reliance on the taxes raised by a duty on the 'remedies'.

Many of the cases reported suggest that it was the poor who were most vulnerable to the dangers of self-diagnosis and treatment with proprietary medicines.

The *Evening Standard* of 12 November 1845 reported on another case involving a child, Matthew Muir, whose death was caused by the effects of 'sugar of lead' which had caused 'paralysis of the involuntary muscles, general emaciation and depraved condition of the blood'. The mixture had been prepared by a Mr Gibbons of Shoreditch 'who sold it to the poor to treat whooping-cough'. Analysis at The London Hospital had shown the mixture contained enough to poison the 5-year-old. Poor Matthew has been dosed on this medicine for about six weeks, and despite the fact that Gibbons had given instructions on the label that a laxative should be administered at the same time, most, including castor oil, would have had no effect. The parents were exonerated, and the court concluded that a verdict of manslaughter would be difficult to prove. Other people came forward to say how beneficial they had found Gibbons' medicine to be, and the jury found it hard to come to a verdict, with some considering the medicine so dangerous it should be withdrawn, and others thinking that Gibbons simply needed to make the instructions on the bottle clearer (despite this being at a time when many of the poor could still not read). The coroner stated that if another case should come before him, Gibbons would be held responsible, but held that Matthew's death to be 'natural'. Gibbons withdrew his medicine.

The year before, in October 1844, a case came before the Westminster Coroner's Court, where the coroner, Mr Higgs, heard the tragic tale of an unnamed 9-week-old child who had died, seemingly due to the ingestion of a 'Godfrey's Cordial', administered by its desperate father. The cordial was a quack medicine 'composed of laudanum and treacle', apparently used by mothers who had no idea that it was dangerous to infants. The coroner observed that 'he scarcely knew any medicine which had so large a sale; he knew of one man alone who sold gallons of it in a single week and realised a handsome fortune in a short space of time'.

It transpired that the family was in dire need of assistance, owing to the husband being out of work, but had been neglected by the parish. The child had not been visited as often by the surgeon as was necessary – Mr Lovett, medical officer of the union, had not visited on a Sunday, and his assistant had given an emetic, despite the fact that he knew it would do no good. Lovett and his assistant were adamant that the proper care had been given, but the report suggests that the surgeon had already decided it was a hopeless case, even before the child was born, openly saying that 'he was convinced that the child could not live, as from the destitute state of the mother, she was unable to afford it the proper nutriment'. This was supported by Mr Jemmett, a physician at King's College Hospital, who had undertaken a post mortem and noted the 'dreadfully emaciated appearance' of the child, who had died of starvation. The father was not to blame, and the full weight of the court's ire came down on the medical officers of the parish.

The jury was horrified. The fact that the mother could not feed the child herself made intervention even more important. The foreman is reported as saying: 'I think this is the most shameful case of neglect. Had it been the case of a rich person, instead of persons wanting the common necessaries of life, the surgeon would have attended on Sunday and the result might have been very different.'

However, these entrepreneurial salespeople existed in, and treated, even the most aristocratic circles and 'quack' medicines were used to treat patients by some of the most famous doctors in the biggest London hospitals. It was unsurprising that they were still so popular with such open endorsement.

In the 1830s Thomas Wakley established the 'Anti-medical Quackery Society' to 'educate the public and to ensure the total suppression of the sale of stamped patent and secret medicines'. Roy Porter describes Wakley as 'at times messianic' in his zeal and determination to end quackery in 'high places'. However, his campaign was always to be frustrated by the simple fact that even the most famous of doctors were endorsing products that were of no proven worth. These arguments took place at a time of great medical advances, but medical treatment and cure were still in their infancy. Many of the preparations offered by general practitioners working across the country were of dubious worth (see Chapter 5). Who, the argument ran, was to say what was 'quack' and what was not? Even after exposure, the famous doctors, such as a surgeon to Guy's Hospital, Bransby Cooper, exposed by *The Lancet*, had no fear of punishment at the hand of the medical colleges.

Roy Porter points out, and Caroline Rance on thequackdoctor.com website, and in her book of the same name (*The Quack Doctor: Historical Remedies for all your Ills*) illustrates in detail, that despite Wakley's best efforts, with the advent of Queen Victoria's reign, the patent medicine market was huge and continued to flourish throughout the nineteenth century and on into the twentieth, when the National Health Service and antibiotics gave everyone access to treatments that could cure and treat symptoms rather than mask them at best and, in the case of the worst of them, cause additional, possibly fatal, results after taking them.

Chapter 7

'His genius gain'd such trust…'
some good men of their time

The title of this chapter is taken from a poem written by a grateful patient to Dr Henry Jephson, famous in his hometown of Leamington Spa, but little known outside it. This is true of most of the men in the next two chapters. Some work has been done on uncovering their lives, usually as part of post-graduate study or as family history. We know as much as we do about Robert Storrs, for example, because of the fine work undertaken by John Tooth, Storrs's great-great-grandson, to bring his archive together, publishing a book and depositing his papers at the Wellcome Library, where hours can be spent amongst his diaries and papers. Henry Stephens is (slightly) more famous as the creator of Stephens' Ink than as the surgeon-apothecary he was. He shared digs with the poet John Keats at Guy's Hospital as they both trained as surgeon-apothecaries in 1815, and is the source of some famous, if rather sniping, anecdotes about the poet. Charles Turner Thackrah is known as one of the founders of occupational medicine and was a co-founder of the Leeds medical school. His life shares some parallels with that of Keats, not least because of his early death, and Thomas Paytherus, who was a close friend and helper to Edward Jenner, pioneer of the smallpox vaccine. Lastly, there is James Parkinson, who was the first to write up the symptoms of what he called 'shaking palsy', his work was later confirmed by other doctors and renamed 'Parkinson's Disease'. His life is a fascinating one, combining as it does radicalism, medicine, and palaeontology.

These men are not just interesting in their own right. Their lives, their training and their experience in the practice offer a more detailed picture of the life led by many of such men, now lost to history, who worked hard to do as much for their patients as they could, often within very limited means, and strove to make a mark on their medical world.

Robert Storrs – A Doncaster medical man who saved the lives of thousands

Robert Storrs was born in Doncaster on 23 June 1801, the only child of John and Elizabeth Storrs. Sadly, he was to lose his mother just two years later, and John was left to bring up the child by himself.

We know a lot about the life of Robert Storrs, owing to the work undertaken by John Tooth, his great-great-grandson, who wrote the book *Human and Heroic: the life and love of a 19th-century doctor* (published privately) largely for the family record. However, his detailed research offers some great insights not just into the life of his forebears, but also gives us a picture of the life led by many a newly qualified surgeon–apothecary (or general practitioner) just after the enactment of the Apothecaries Act 1815.

Even John Tooth's diligent investigation has not been able to uncover any real detail about Storrs's early life, apart from the mentions he made of it in letters to his wife in later years. He wrote of lonely times, without the comfort of parental affection and there is little evidence of who gave him the most support during his childhood. After the death of his mother, his father, John, employed a housekeeper, Charlotte Robinson, who bore him a daughter, Anne, when Robert was already 18 and just coming to the end of his apprenticeship. Although it is likely he had made good progress at the local grammar school (where he was known to be intelligent, and keen to experiment with poetry), he left his schooling aged about 15 and was apprenticed to a local surgeon, Mr Moore, and an apothecary, Mr Popplewell. The exact term he would serve under Moore and Popplewell is unknown, as is the premium, although at this time it was likely to be around £150 to £200.

To practise as a surgeon–apothecary Storrs needed, after 1815, to obtain the Licentiate of the Society of Apothecaries and be accepted as a Member of the Royal College of Surgeons. Working as a provincial doctor, he would then be qualified to treat disease and injury and prescribe and make his own medicines.

Like many other young men mentioned in this book, Storrs chose to move to London to attend the lectures and gain the necessary hands-on hospital experience in preparation for the examinations he must take to complete his training. Like John Keats and Henry Stephens before him, he enrolled at Guy's Hospital, probably leaving Doncaster around 22 August 1822, and, like Keats and Stephens, he was lucky enough to study under the great surgeon Sir Astley Cooper who was at that time in his prime, and one of the highest paid professional men in Europe, earning more than £20,000 per annum. Recently knighted by King George IV after removing a cyst from his scalp, he was known to be a compassionate man, idolised by his students, and someone who still treated even the poorest patients at the hospital with respect. John Tooth points out that Robert was keen to behave to his own patients as Astley did to his, and was well known for his 'courtesy and dedication' to all in his care.

Robert studied hard at Guy's, preparing four papers which he presented to the prestigious Guy's Hospital Physical Society, but like all other would-be doctors he also had to take on the responsibility of walking the wards with the senior doctors, perhaps dressing wounds and undertaking minor procedures such as lancing a boil, as directed. He was also required to dissect the bodies and diseased organs available to students in the dissection room. These bodies were rarely fresh and could well have been provided by the services of the 'resurrection men' or body snatchers, working in the nearby cemeteries. (See Chapter 3.)

Robert Storrs was an ambitious young man, and passed the necessary exams, leaving Guy's Hospital and returning to Doncaster in the spring of 1824. He needed to establish himself quickly because, late in his studies, he met his wife to be, Martha 'Patty' Townsend at a party, and her family would not have been keen to see her commit herself to a surgeon–apothecary of small means. At this time, the social standing of a surgeon–apothecary was still in some doubt. Was he a gentleman? Or was he 'trade'? With whom was it proper for him to dine? The class structure of the medical world had, for years, seen only the university trained 'physician' dining with his wealthy patients, despite the fact that their medical knowledge may not be as practical and up to date as the surgeon. The apothecary was seen by many to be a mere shopkeeper, however, and it was some time before the distinctions became sufficiently blurred to admit any but the most celebrated general doctor into fashionable society.

Welcomed back into the bosom of his family after a gruelling journey back to Doncaster, he took steps to contact his old mentor, Mr Moore, who was still a popular surgeon in the town. However, the terms upon which Moore would do business were not acceptable to Storrs and he decided to establish his own practice – a very brave step at that time. It offered no steady income and required him to work in competition with many other, more well-established, doctors in the area. However, Storrs considered it to be the best way forward and in July 1824 he placed an advertisement in *The Doncaster, Nottingham and Lincoln Gazette* that read:

R.Storrs

Member of the Royal College of Surgeons in London
and Licentiate of the Worshipful Company of Apothecaries,
RESPECTFULLY announces to his Friends and
the Public, that he intends PRACTISING the
Various branches of the Profession, in Doncaster and
its Vicinity, and trusts his attention and assiduity will
merit some share of the public patronage and support.
R.S. has paid particular attention to the Diseases
of the eye, at the London Ophthalmic Infirmary.
Miss Fletcher's, French gate
Doncaster, July 1st 1824

(Source: *Heroic and Humane*)

Luckily for researchers, Robert Storrs decided early in his new career to start recording his most interesting cases in leather-bound volumes, which have been lodged by his family at the Wellcome Library in London. In them, he writes detailed medical notes of the treatments he prescribed and the outcome of his endeavours. For detail of the cases Storrs and his contemporaries dealt with, and the success or otherwise of the options available to cure or alleviate suffering, see Chapter 5. It is true from some of the reports Storrs makes that it was somewhat easier for a surgeon-apothecary of the time to succeed with a surgical intervention, than with a medical one. There were so few medicines available, no antibiotics for example, and equipment available in top London hospitals (stethoscopes perhaps) was rarely available to the small town doctor at this time. There were no X-rays or other diagnostic tests so usually all the doctor could do was bleed or purge, often to the patient's detriment rather than cure.

By the beginning of 1825, Storrs was seeing some growth in his practice, but it is a sign of the difficulties faced by new young general practitioners at this time, that his income was still not considered sufficient to support a wife. His romance with Martha Townsend had continued unabated, but only by letter; Storrs was not a regular visitor to London and it was not until 1827 that they were able to marry. Martha was just 19, and it would have been a significant step for her to move away from her family to support her husband back in Doncaster.

Robert Storrs's notebooks and his letters to Martha offer a wonderful picture of small-town life in the early nineteenth century, but more than that they are in themselves a social history of medicine at the time. In many of Storrs notes, his treatment of patients would seem wrong today. He was not alone in having to face life-threatening illness with very few tools at his disposal. His treatment of patients during a cholera outbreak in the town, for example, highlights how little the medical establishment knew of the way in which the disease was spread. He says in his notes: 'I feel almost as much in the dark as previous to the commencement of the disease in this town…'

He goes on to describe in some detail the treatments that the poor souls, already in agony with the symptoms of the disease – the vomiting and diarrhoea, cramps and dehydration – were given in an attempt to rid them of the 'poison', as Storrs describes it. It is Storrs's notebooks that offer a provincial doctor's view of the causes of, and treatments suitable for, many of the conditions identified. What is clear from Storrs's words is that he is desperate to find some means of improving the lot of his patients, even when they are clearly in the final stages of something as virulent as cholera.

But it is perhaps the work done by Robert Storrs in the field of obstetrics, and more specifically in his observations on the causes of 'childbed', or puerperal fever, that should have cemented his place in the history of medicine. For many years, a Hungarian obstetrician called Ignaz Semmelweis was credited with having recognised the importance of good hygiene to avoid cross-contamination of patients, most particularly after childbirth. John Tooth, in *Humane and Heroic*, suggests that had Storrs been practising in a major centre, such as London, then his work on the subject would have been given prominence. His writings on the subject, in a paper for *The Provincial Medical Journal*, were published some seven years before Semmelweis's work came to prominence. As it was, it took until 2005, and the work of Dr Milton Wainwright from the University of Sheffield's Department of Molecular Biology and Biotechnology, to highlight Storrs's role in saving the lives of many otherwise vulnerable mothers.

Storrs had become concerned when he was involved in a series of births in which the women had contracted a puerperal fever, eight of whom had died. He researched the matter exhaustively and began to notice the possible influence of factors outside of childbirth itself. He had already noted that during the period when so many women had died, there were also outbreaks of typhus, scarlatina and erysipelas in Doncaster, and he came to believe that some form of contamination from the erysipelas had reached the women's genital tracts. He had reached this conclusion despite the fact that there was no knowledge of the action of bacteria and viruses at the time, and his acknowledgement that he must have carried the 'poison' from one patient to another, thus infecting the women with it, caused him significant anxiety and pain:

> *I attended on the 22nd and the 24th three other cases of midwifery, having made every possible ablution and in an entire change of clothes,; all the patients did well but considering that it would be too great a risk to continue to do so after producing such a great amount of misery, I determined I would attend no more for some time...*

Storrs was certainly not alone in spreading the infection in this way, but many doctors still disputed that they might have been the cause of 'such a great amount of misery'. However, Storrs found support amongst many doctors in his local area, and his new methods to prevent the cross-contamination must have saved many lives, especially as he went on to address audiences on the importance of cleanliness not only in the birth room but elsewhere too, acknowledging that if erysipelas could spread from patient to patient, then it was likely that other such conditions could be spread from person to person too.

Dr Milton Wainwright is quoted as saying: 'Thanks to pioneers like Doncaster's Dr Storrs we now know that good hygiene is vital and doctors and nurses, in particular, are encouraged to thoroughly wash their hands to prevent the spread of infection.'

The fine work undertaken by this most dedicated of practitioners is ultimately deeply ironic. When the famine in Ireland resulted in the immigration of starving Irish families, Robert Storrs was one of the few doctors willing to nurse them when they contracted typhus, something to which they were particularly vulnerable in their state of health and the unsanitary conditions in which they had to live. As John Tooth says, Robert Storrs would have been unaware of the risks he was taking when treating patients in the Union Workhouse, as the cause (the excreta of a louse) was then unknown. Sadly, he contracted typhus and died, three weeks later, on 14 September 1847, aged just 46.

Obituaries in the local press were glowing, recognising the work he had done and the sacrifice he had made 'on the field of duty, and he goes to the grave with a character esteemed and respected by thousands'. The papers drew attention to his heartbroken wife, Martha, and the twelve children the couple had together.

The untiring energy of his professional character was not more remarkable than his suavity of manners and gentleness of disposition, which endeared his memory to the heart of his townsmen.

Henry Jephson – 'Remarkable physician and philanthropist'

Born in Sutton-in-Ashfield in Nottinghamshire on 4 October 1798, Henry Jephson was the sixth in a family of eight boys. He lived with his mother, Mary, and his father, Richard Jephson, who was a skilled artisan, a 'framesmith', who made and repaired the frames constructed to produce stockings. Although there is no specific detail available, as a child, Henry would have been living through dangerous times, his father being involved in a trade subject to economic depression and the actions of the Luddites.

In late 1812 or early 1813, the 14-year-old Henry took up an apprenticeship with a Mr Henry Clowishaw of Mansfield in Nottinghamshire. Sadly, records at the Society of Apothecaries do not give the date of his first steps towards a medical career, nor is the premium his parents would have had to pay given, although the figure was commonly around £200. Later, Jephson was to remark that this was, financially, a very challenging period in his life. His parents were not wealthy, and with eight boys to educate there was little enough to go round.

Eric Baxter, in his book *Dr Jephson of Leamington Spa* suggests it is probable that after completing his apprenticeship Henry continued his medical studies in London, and indeed he later recalled that he had come to Leamington Spa on the recommendation of one of his tutors, after a period of ill health (due to a period of desperate poverty). He interrupted his medical studies to take a place at the surgery of a Mr Chambers, one of the first surgeons to establish himself in Leamington Spa, who was himself unwell and who had advertised for someone to assist him while he recovered.

Leamington Spa appeared to suit Jephson, as he remained working with Chambers's expanding practice until 1822 when he decided to resume his studies in London to become qualified and establish his professional status. He enrolled at the Middlesex Hospital in London on 21 September 1822 and at St George's in October the same year. In both hospitals he was under the tutelage of distinguished medical men: the physician Dr William

MacMichael and surgeon Mr (later Sir) Benjamin Brodie. Records show that he qualified as Licentiate of the Society of Apothecaries in May 1923, and on his return to Leamington was to be taken into partnership with Chambers, as a surgeon–apothecary.

By this time Chambers was surgeon to some very influential people, such as the Duke of Clarence (he was later to become Surgeon Extraordinary to William IV) and Jephson made some important connections that would serve him well later in his career. Also around this time, he met his future wife, Ann Eliza Geldart.

Henry's partnership with Chambers was dissolved in 1827, possibly because Jephson was becoming the more popular of the two men; later in that year and into 1828, he was in Glasgow to qualify as a Doctor of Medicine, before returning to Leamington to establish his own practice in the town. Buoyed up by the knowledge that his popularity with his patients, already evident before he completed his studies, had resulted in his fame spreading well outside the boundaries of the town, he took one of the large terraced houses in the then fashionable York Terrace and his list of patients quickly increased, to include members of all the armed forces, men of government and their families and even patients from abroad who would stay at the Regent Hotel in order to seek his advice.

Letters and diaries of the rich and famous, as well as Jephson's own records and subscriptions for his engraved portraits, indicate his list could almost be a 'who's who' of important people from the 1820s to the middle of the nineteenth century. The sixth son of an artisan had not found his humble beginnings to be any handicap in a career that saw him treat Viscount and Viscountess Sidmouth, the Dowager Marchioness of Queensberry, and the Earl of Wemyss for example. Others who mention him in their papers include art critic John Ruskin, the clown Joseph Grimaldi, and Florence Nightingales's mother and sister, Fanny and Parthenope Nightingale. It was also rumoured that Jephson treated the young Queen Victoria.

It is worth noting at this point that the 'Leamington Priors mineral springs' had been promoted as 'health giving' by local doctors from the 1700s onwards, although it wasn't until around Jephson's time that they were commercially exploited. Like similar spa resorts, such as Bath, the drinking of the supposedly health-giving mineral waters, and also regular bathing in them, was marketed as 'taking the waters', with much of the advertising undertaken by the local medical community.

There are some details of Jephson's treatments available that indicate he was much sought after for upset stomachs, dyspepsia, obesity, mild heart conditions, and nervous exhaustion. A letter sent to a Colonel Newdigate, Dartmouth Road, Blackheath on 14 August 1837 reads:

My dear Sir,

I recommend you use a tepid shower bath every morning with your head covered and your feet placed in water, and to take the mixture and pills prescribed for four or five weeks.

You must vary the dose of the pills according to the effects they produce upon your bowels.

Walk for an hour before each meal.

Live upon plain meat, poultry, game, mealy potatoes, stale bread, plain puddings, eggs lightly oiled, sherry, toast and water, black tea and butter only.

With my kind wishes

Henry Jephson

Reports suggest he was something of a 'benevolent despot' who might take a ride in a carriage with a patient, only to set them down and tell them to walk home (for the exercise). He was also known to turn up unexpectedly as his patients' residences at mealtimes to ascertain whether banned luxuries were being consumed, thereby affecting his cure rate and ultimately his reputation. Certainly, his diagnoses and treatment regime were successful, perhaps partly because many of those who came to him were suffering from nothing more serious than over-indulgence and indigestion.

His home in York Terrace was soon found to be too small, although it was his patients and the entertaining of them that made it so because, sadly, he and his wife had just one child, who had died in infancy. His income was now increasing as rapidly as his list, and so he decided to build a new home, a mansion in Warwick Street, Leamington Spa, known as Beech Lawn. When it was completed in 1832, its value was assessed at £125 (more than £5,000 in today's money) – a figure that seems more remarkable when it is compared to other great properties of the time. It was worth more than the Royal Pump Room and Baths, and £40 more than the Bath Hotel, and had a double drawing room, large dining room, library, consulting room and fourteen bedrooms, as well as a number of rooms for staff and extensive cellars. It enjoyed a position in three acres of land and had extensive gardens and greenhouses, as well as a coach house for three coaches and five horses. Jephson lived at Beech Lawn for the rest of his life. The property was demolished in 1946, but not before it had been divided and its land sold for housing and the house and some grounds turned into a girls' school. It is now the site of the local fire station.

His practice at Beech Lawn continued to expand and the doctor was lauded locally as a man who brought significant trade to the rest of Leamington Spa. His own salary grew exponentially and contemporaries called his income 'almost fabulous'. It is certain that for many years he earned in excess of £20,000 and there is little doubt that, in twenty-first-century terms, he was a millionaire. Part of Jephson's appeal, however, and his longevity as one of the great and good of the town is based on his reputation as a philanthropist.

During the 1830s and 40s it is thought that Jephson set aside as much as two hours of each morning to treat the poor of the town, and if he earned anything from richer clients on a Sunday, the money would be distributed amongst those same poor patients. He researched the issue of deficient sewerage in the area and engaged the experts necessary to address it. Many of the facilities enjoyed by all in the town of Leamington Spa had been provided by generous donations from Jephson and supported individuals in need. It was said of him that 'Jephson made Leamington and Leamington made Jephson', and a jingle composed at the time went:

> *You knew that Dr Jephson! Well rather,*
> *And perhaps you will not say ah!*
> *If I add he was Leamington's father,*
> *Or that in fact, he was Leamington' S-pa*

He gave regularly to the local church funds and supported the foundation of Leamington College for Boys, and served as both magistrate and vice-president and governor of the Leamington's Warneford Hospital.

The public was keen to show their appreciation of the good doctor, and presentations were made 'in testimony of your high medical skill, your humanity to the afflicted poor and your unwearied perseverance in promoting the interests of the town of Leamington'.

Eric Baxter in *Dr Jephson of Leamington Spa* recounts an incident when, after a month away for his own health in the German town of Baden-Baden, he returned to 'several enlivening peals' rung at the parish church, and was presented with a petition asking him not to go away again as the place became deserted in his absence.

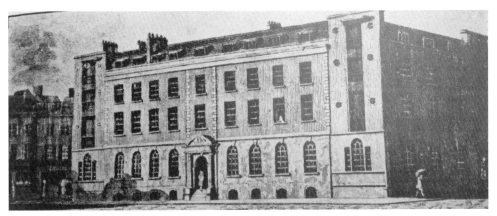

The Apothecaries Hall, eighteenth century.

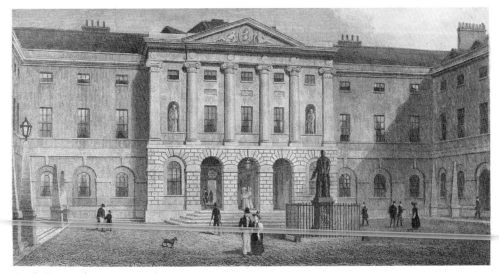

Guy's Hospital in 1831. *(Wellcome Library)*

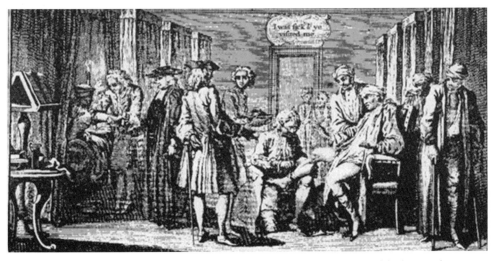

The City Infirmary, Northampton was an early hospital, founded by Dr Doddridge & others, 1743.

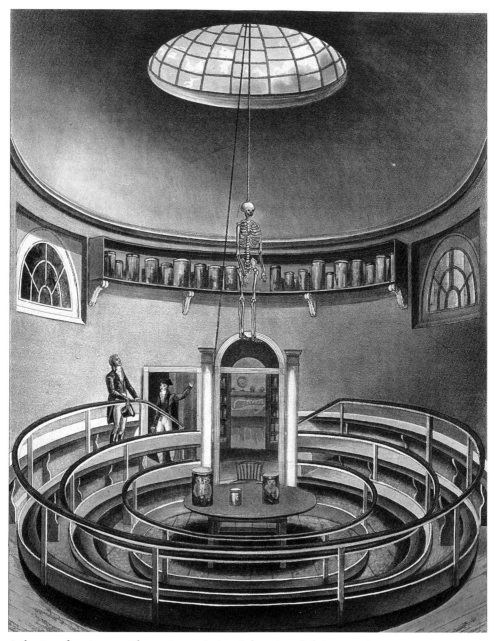

A theatre of anatomy, with specimens in jars & hanging skeleton. *(Wellcome Library)*

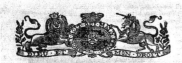

ANNO QUINQUAGESIMO QUINTO

GEORGII III. REGIS.

✦✦✦

C A P. CXCIV.

An Act for better regulating the Practice of Apothecaries throughout *England* and *Wales*.

[12th *July* 1815.]

WHEREAS His Majesty King *James* the First, by Letters Patent, under the Great Seal of *Great Britain*, bearing Date the Sixth Day of *December*, in the Fifteenth Year of His Reign, did for Himself, His Heirs and Successors, grant unto *William Besse*, and divers other Persons therein named, and to all and singular other Persons whomsoever, brought up and skilful in the Art, Mystery, or Faculty of Apothecaries, and exercising the same Art, Mystery, or Faculty, then being Freemen of the Mystery of Grocers of the City of *London*, or being Freemen of any other Art, Mystery, or Faculty in the said City of *London* (so as they had been brought up and were expert in the Art or Mystery of Apothecaries), that they, and all such Men of the said Art or Mystery of Apothecaries of and in the said City of *London* and Suburbs of the same, and within Seven Miles of the said City, might and should be one Body Corporate and Politic, in Substance, Deed, and Name, by the Name of the Master, Wardens, and Society of the Art and Mystery of Apothecaries of the City of *London*; and did ordain and declare, that by the same Name they might have perpetual Succession, and have, purchase, possess, enjoy, and retain Manors, Messuages, Lands, Tenements, Liberties, Privileges, Franchises, Jurisdictions, and Hereditaments to them and their Successors, in Fee Simple and Perpetuity, or for Term of Year or Years, or otherwise howsoever; and also Goods and Chattels, and all

Charter by Jac. 1. to the Apothecaries Company recited.

19 U   other

The Apothecaries Act 1815, a watershed in the training of medical men.

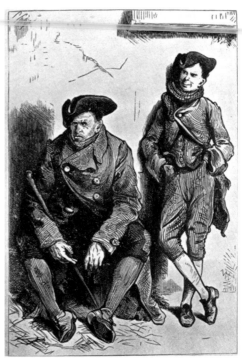

An apothecary in his shop.

'The Resurrectionists'.
(Wellcome Library)

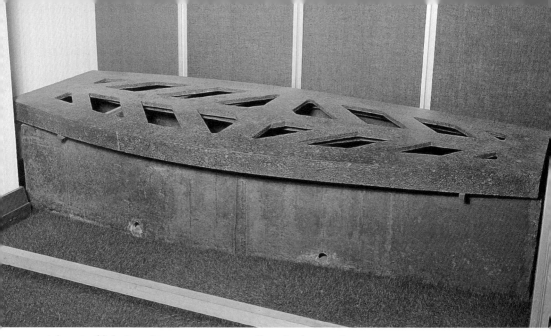

A 'mortsafe' designed to protect a corpse from body-snatchers. *(Wellcome Library)*

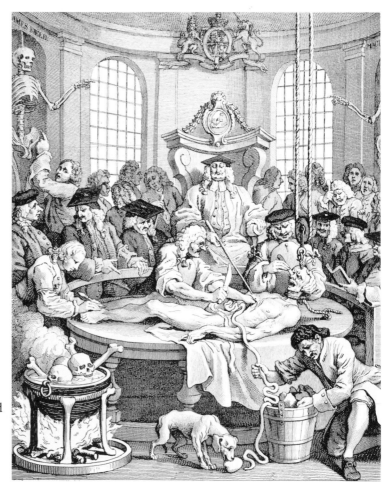

Hogarth's 'The Reward of Crewelty' published in 1851, showing a murderer being hanged and publicly dissected.

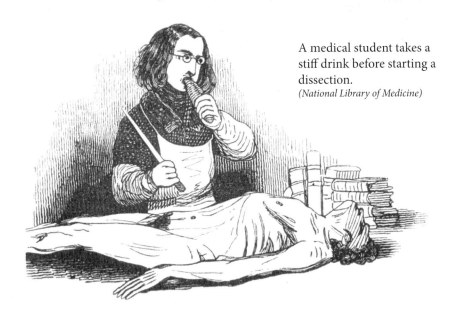

A medical student takes a stiff drink before starting a dissection.
(National Library of Medicine)

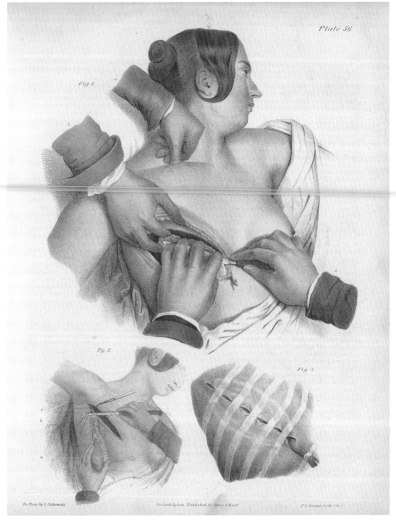

Surgery for the removal of the mammary gland, 1846.
(Wellcome Library)

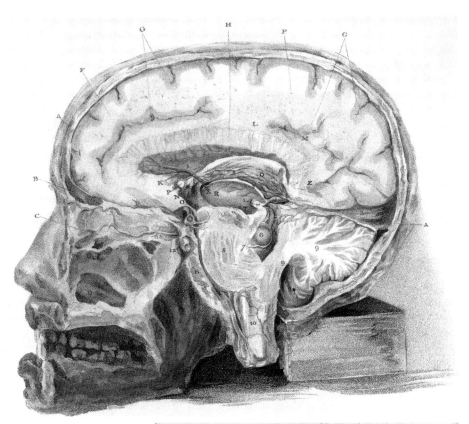

A section of the brain, Sir
Charles Bell, 1802.
(Wellcome Library)

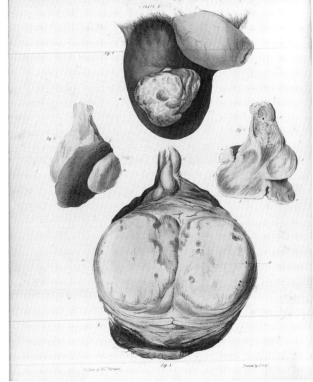

A depiction of a chronic
enlargement of the testis, by Sir
Astley Cooper, 1830.
(Wellcome Library)

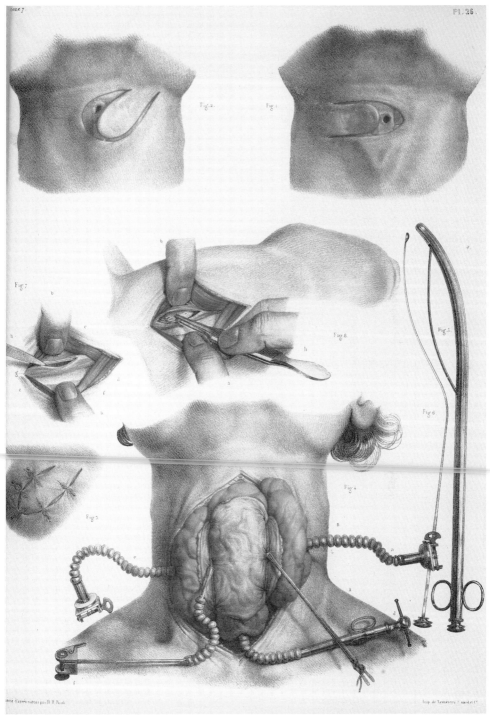

Surgical procedures of the neck. *(National Library of Medicine)*

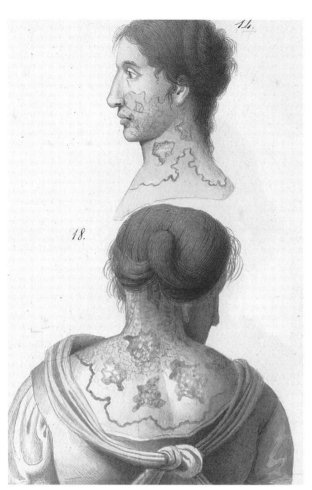

Head and neck of a woman with syphilis. *(National Library of Medicine)*

Comparing two sets of apparatus to splint a broken leg. J. Bell, 1802. *(Wellcome Library)*

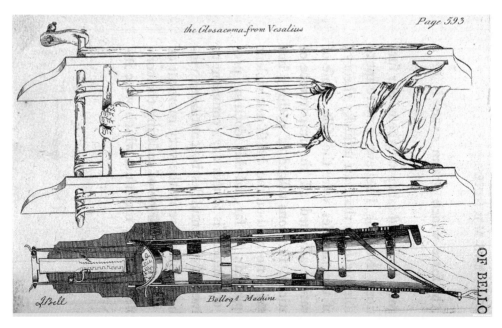

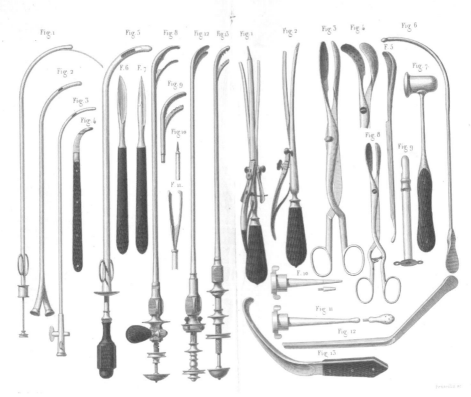

Surgical instruments used in the removal of a kidney or bladder stone (lithotripsy), 1848.
(Wellcome Library)

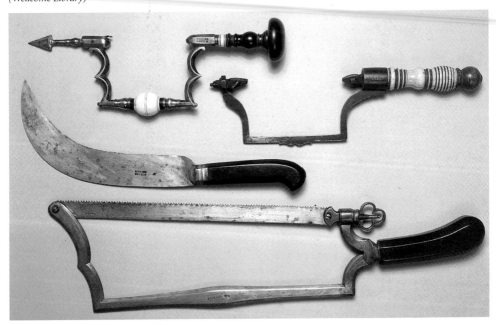

Amputation instruments and apparatus. *(Wellcome Library)*

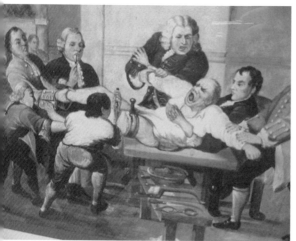

An amputation, before anaesthetic.

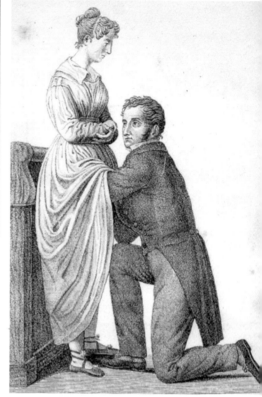

The internal examination of a woman.
(janeaustensworld.wordpress.com)

Three heads illustrating different methods of bandaging. J. Bell, early nineteenth century.
(Wellcome Library)

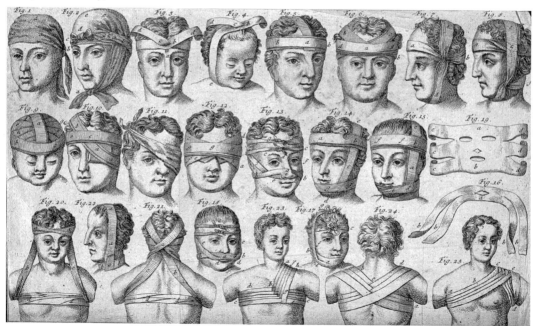

A surgeon's tools for childbirth, eighteenth century. *(Wellcome Library)*

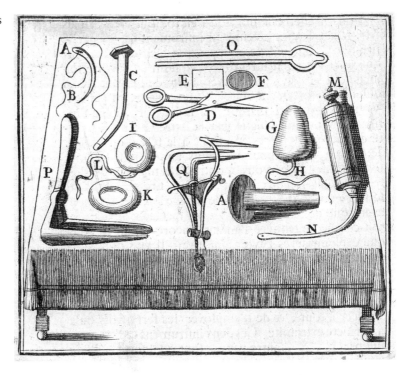

A birth scene by an unknown French artist, 1800. *(Wellcome Library)*

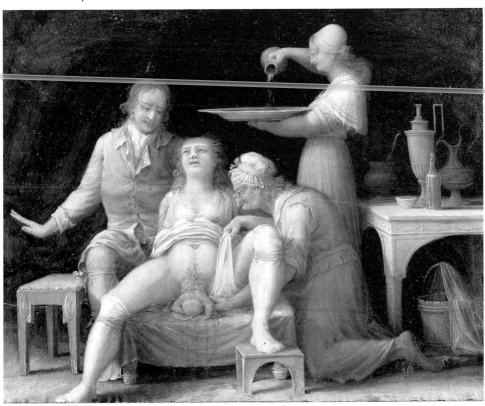

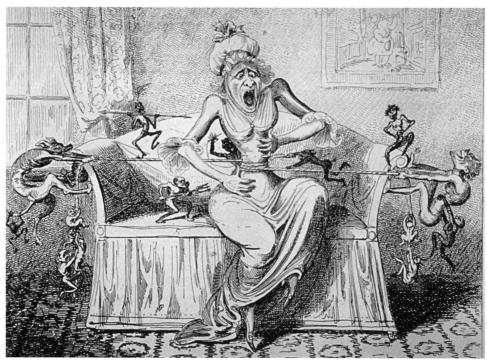

'The Cholic' cartoon by George Cruickshank, illustrating the pain of digestive problems.

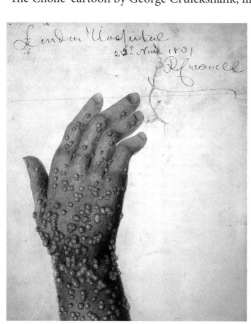

Green Smallpox pustules, by Carswell.
(Wellcome Library)

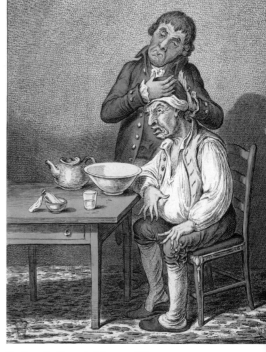

'A Gentle Emetic', James Gilray.
(The British Museum)

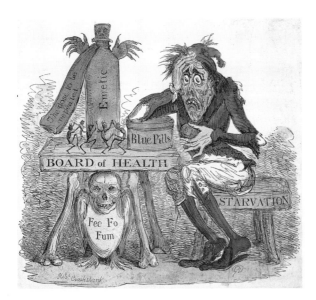

A cholera patient experimenting with (useless) remedies, by Robert Cruickshank. *(Wellcome Library)*

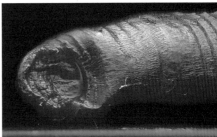

Mouthparts of a medicinal leech. *(Wellcome Library)*

Surging letting blood from a woman's arm, eighteenth century. *(Wellcome Library)*

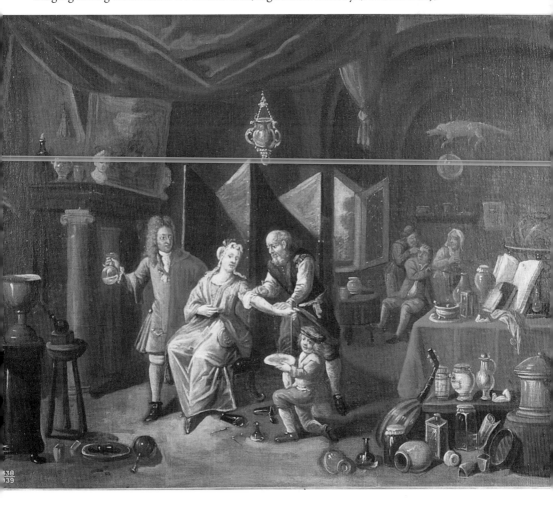

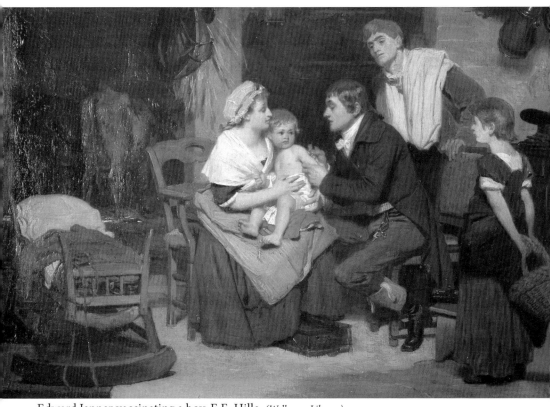

Edward Jenner vaccinating a boy. E.E. Hille. *(Wellcome Library)*

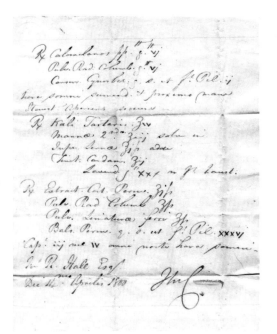

Prescription for Richard Hall, Georgian Gentleman. *(Mike Rendell)*

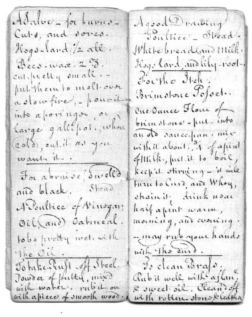

Eighteenth-century home medical recipe book kept by Richard Hall. *(Mike Rendell)*

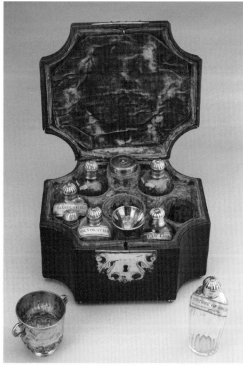

Eighteenth-century medicine chest. *(Science Museum)*

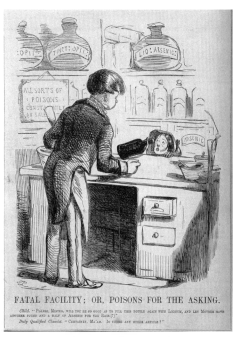

An unscrupulous apothecary selling arsenic and laudanum to a child. *(Wellcome Library)*

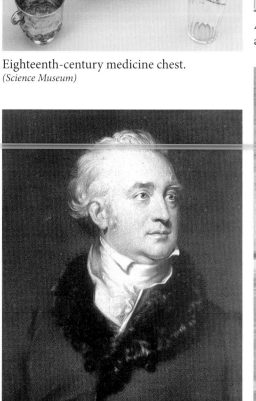

Sir Astley Cooper. *(Wellcome Library)*

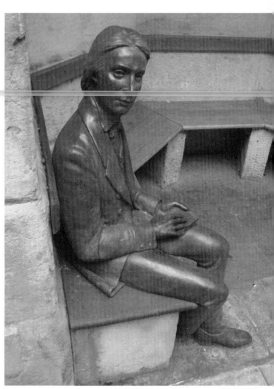

Statue of John Keats at Guy's Hospital, London. *(Mike Paterson)*

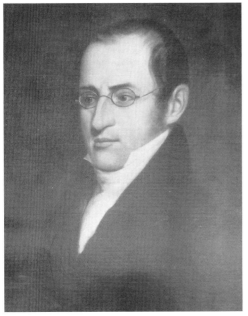

Charles Turner Thackrah.

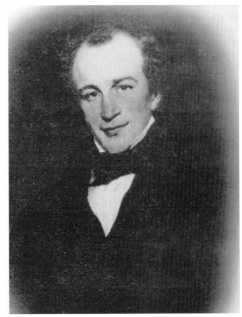

Robert Storrs. *(John Tooth)*

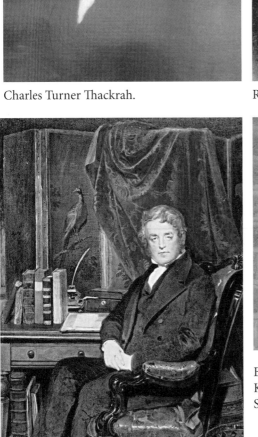

Henry Jephson, by John Bostock, June 1850.
(Leamington Spa History Group)

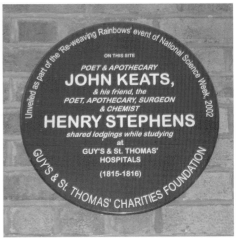

Blue plaque on the lodgings shared by John Keats and Henry Stephens, 3 St. Thomas' Street, Southwark.

Those who had been treated by Jephson were moved to write poetry to him. Maria Jane Jewsbury wrote a 'Winter welcomed', and in December 1846 the following appeared in the Leamington Spa Courier, written by one Isabella Graham Fullerton:

To thee with lingering hope the frail and fading flowers we bring
That wear the wintry hue of death in life's unclosing spring
And when its primal bloom again the wasted cheek had won
How marvel that they turn to thee, as spring flowers to the sun?

Steadfast through life's vicissitudes thou art no summer-friend
Whose friendship lasts through pleasant hours, but ends when pleasures end
Thou in the dim and quiet room art yet a willing guest
'Tis from the restless pillow that thy soothing voice is blest.

The homage continues, through another four verses, to the last two, which suggest that to Jephson, the physical memorials were of less value than the gratitude of his patients:

O, what to thee is marble pile, or monumental stone!
The kindling eye, the fluent lip, thy attributes make known
Thy living trophies breathe around, and plead that one so dear
May see a cloudless sun arise on many a coming year

Yet great as is thy mission, great and rare should be thy mead
One by which future ages with no doubting glance may read
'His goodness claim'd such reverence; His genius gain'd such trust
That unto living worth for once this jealous world was just.

The greatest honour bestowed him, however (he apparently turned down a baronetcy more than once, probably because he had no heir) was when a testimonial scheme raised a significant amount of money and it was agreed that the former Newbold Gardens be leased in perpetuity and re-named the Jephson Gardens, and include a specially commissioned temple and statue of Jephson. Whilst recognising their benefactor, it also benefited the town as a whole, a grand dinner was held to celebrate the opening and a specially minted medal was struck to show Jephson on one side and his home, Beech Lawn, on the other.

Despite all the cures he had effected for others, Jephson was unable to ensure his own health. Just two years after the opening of the gardens, and before the statue and temple were completed, it became clear that Dr Henry Jephson would have to retire from his professional practice. He was just 50 years of age, but he had gone blind.

Jephson did not detach himself from the needs of the town, however. He continued to live at Beech Lawn, with his wife and contributed to many local and national appeals for support. His importance to the town diminished of course, as the number of famous guests seeking his medical advice declined, and in the 1860s he was quick to step in when the future of the Pump Rooms was threatened due to a decline in the fashion of 'taking the waters'.

Henry's wife Eliza died in 1874, but he continued to live in the big house, cared for by the children of his brother, William. He lived for a further four years, until, on 1 May 1878, he died from 'failure of nervous power, probably dependent on degeneration of the nerve structure'. The family asked for a quiet funeral, so there was no procession (although there surely would have been), but it is said that many of the biggest tradespeople closed for the duration of the ceremony in the churchyard of St James, Old Milverton, where he was laid to rest with his wife and her sister.

The importance of Henry Jephson lies not with his groundbreaking treatments, but more with, according to Eric Baxter, 'the scale of his success, unprecedented before him and perhaps still unequalled'. His impact on the town of Leamington Spa is undisputed, and his name is still well known in the area, and the gardens remain dedicated to him. In this book, there are men who made more impact on the development of medical treatments, but none who had such influence over the rich and famous of the day.

James Parkinson, General Practitioner – from palsy to palaeontology

James Parkinson is not a man about whom we know very much, but he stands out as a name we now associate with one of the most disabling of progressive neurological conditions – Parkinson's disease (now known more simply as Parkinson's). He was truly a man of science, who first identified and described the illness as 'shaking palsy' in a paper published in 1817. He was also a one-time anti-government pamphleteer and later contributed to the study of palaeontology, being a founder member of the Geological Society. In 1794 he was examined, on oath, by the Privy Council, in relation to a possible connection with the notorious 'pop gun plot' – an alleged conspiracy to assassinate George III with a poisoned dart. Parkinson was, at the time, known as a radical intellectual committed to the reduction of social inequality and as a member of the radical discussion group, The London Corresponding Society, he found himself implicated in the plot. Dr Gerald Stern, in his introduction to the book *Parkinson's Disease*, edited and published in 1990, suggests that it was this 'scare' that discouraged Parkinson from further involvement in the radical movement of the time: 'He ceased to write pamphlets and directed his energies towards matters scientific and medical'.

However, for the purposes of this book, it is his life as a doctor and his writings on the training of, and the life lived by, an effective practitioner that are of greatest interest. His work as surgeon and apothecary in Hoxton over many decades identifies him as one of the original 'General Practitioners'.

Little is known about James Parkinson's early life, although research into his background was undertaken in 1912 by Leonard Rowntree of the John Hopkins Medical School in Baltimore. James William Keys Parkinson was born in 1755 in Hoxton, then a village in the county of Middlesex. Just of the north of the City of London, Hoxton was attractive and genteel, despite having a history of violence and associations with the theatre. In fact, the Square in which the Parkinson family lived was built on a field in which a fatal duel had taken place between Ben Jonson and a fellow actor.

James was the son of John Parkinson, also a doctor, who lived and worked in the area. The house occupied by the family in Hoxton Square was, with the rest of the village, gradually consumed by the needs of the capital as the industrial revolution accelerated. The Square became the centre of the furniture trade; workshops were constructed in the gardens of this once upmarket residential area and by the 1800s it was becoming a densely populated and ultimately deprived part of London, rife with slums. James remained in the area for much of his life, and would have seen many changes; not least the loss of the fields and agricultural land that had surrounded that part of the city. The house in which he lived and practised, at no.1 Hoxton Square, is no longer standing, but the spot is marked by a blue plaque celebrating his achievements.

At the age of 21, probably after years of observation and interest in his father's work, James Parkinson took the decision to follow him into medicine and enrolled at the London Hospital in Whitechapel, to the east of Hoxton. Eight years later, just after the death of his father, he was awarded the diploma of the College of Surgeons (before it became the Royal College) and immediately took over his father's practice, one that was to be run by Parkinson for many years; his own son was to work with him and take over the running of the surgery after James Parkinson retired.

Parkinson became a very active member of the London medical community, being elected a fellow of the Medical Society of London in 1787, writing numerous papers and pamphlets, as well as books on medical advice aimed squarely at those who came to him as a general practitioner. Notable amongst his works is *The Hospital Pupil* of 1800 and *The Villager's Friend and Physician* of 1804. *The Hospital Pupil* was written as correspondence between the author, a father considering medicine as a career for his son, and the son himself. It offers James Parkinson's view of the current state of medical training and of the necessity of any man considering a career as a doctor, if the need to earn a living was necessary, to seek training not as an expert physician or surgeon, but as a more general medical man, closer to his own work as a surgeon-apothecary: 'I need hardly repeat to you the vulgar observation that a physician seldom obtains bread by his profession until he has no teeth left to eat it.'

His views on training in medicine are unequivocal – he considers the usual route to be totally inadequate:

> *The first four or five years are almost entirely appropriated to the compounding of medicines, the art of which, with every habit of necessary exactness, might be just as well obtained in as many months.... The remaining years of his apprenticeship bring with them the acquisition of the art of bleeding, of dressing a blister and for the completion of the climax – of exhibiting an enema...*

He considers that, as the next stage is to enter a hospital to attend lectures and to walk the wards to observe more senior doctors at work, this early education is woefully inadequate. He insists a lengthy attendance at lectures on anatomy, physiology, and chemistry would be useful, along with a pleasant side-interest in botany, to ensure that as a student he can make the best of the information imparted to him.

It is interesting to wonder how far the advice offered by Parkinson in his book is gleaned from his own direct experience, either from his own education or from observation of the lack of necessary knowledge obvious in his contemporaries at The London Hospital. Most likely, he was given the opportunity to learn from his father's experience and was offered a good grounding in the subjects he alludes to, as the tone of the pamphlet does not seem to indicate any regret on his part. He moralises, whilst saying he refuses to do so, but his description of student life will be familiar to many more than 200 years later:

An associate invites you to accompany him to the play; but you, knowing you have some evening lecture to attend beg to be excused…. Your objection is opposed by the observation, that 'you really make too much of a slave of yourself…besides our friend here will promise you the loan of his notes of the lecture….' Thus if you are not sufficiently guarded are you enticed into the party; and when you arrive at the play house, are probably joined by the friend on whose notes you depended….

Drunkenness ensues, and so much wine is consumed that morning lectures are also missed. The notes you borrow are poor and thus, maintains Parkinson, begins the journey down the slippery slope: '…and too often will this idea of postponement when once admitted, warp your resolutions of industry, and influence your determinations, when exposed to similar invitations'.

However, the book is not all moralising and careers advice. Towards the end, Parkinson enters into a discussion on the subject of madness with the young would-be doctor. This is an area in which he has some considerable experience, owing to his treatment of patients in the significant number of asylums sited in and around the Hoxton area. It shows him to be an enlightened and empathic man. Here his comments on what we would now consider a case of post-natal depression or psychosis:

I am sure you will oppose the too early removal [to a mental institution] *of females who, unhappily, in a few days after delivering, manifest symptoms of derangement. I have known a removal to a mad-house take place a fortnight after delivery, but surely at that period, such a change can hardly produce any advantages to compensate for a loss of those tender attentions, which the poor unfortunate being might be enabled to receive at her own home…*

In light of the incarceration of women in asylums in the Victorian period, for apparent mental health issues we find impossible to understand today – 'disappointment in love' for example, or being 'argumentative' with, usually male, relations – Parkinson's view is well ahead of his time.

He also entreats the young doctor to deal with those who 'destroy themselves [commit suicide] with mercy', to avoid hurting the innocent relatives left behind. There was an awful stigma to suicide that could leave the family vulnerable to the seizure of their loved one's property unless insanity could be asserted. Thus poverty could only be averted by concerns over the inheritance of madness and it was no wonder so many who could afford to do so tried to cover up a suicide.

I can only entreat you, in every case, where the lives, or the sufferings of your fellow creatures, depend on your opinion, to deliver it with that caution, for which the awfulness of the case calls; and to resolve to promote justice, but incline to mercy.

Perhaps the most telling paragraph comes when he describes what he believes it takes to be a good doctor, and the effects that a wrong career choice can have:

A sympathetic concern, and a tender interest for the sufferings of others, ought to characterize all those who engage themselves in a profession, the object of which should be to mitigate or remove the great portion of the calamities to which humanity is subject. For he, who can view the sufferings of a fellow creature with unconcern, will, there is much to reason the fear, sometimes neglect the opportunities of administering the required relief; that relief which he could with ease bestow, and which he withholds only from his not feeling, with due force, the afflicting urgency of the claim, which is made on him.

In 1804 Parkinson wrote another book offering an insight into his views of his profession. This time he addresses his patients directly in *The Villager's Friend and Physician*, which offers advice on, and details the treatment of, a number of common ailments such as 'quinsy', croup, or gout, and offers descriptions of many of the illnesses that, at the time, regularly proved fatal. He offered suggestions for preventative measures any patient could take, including dietary advice such as avoiding spices and adhering to a rather nauseating healthy eating plan:

He that breakfasts on milk, dines one day on animal food, and the other on pudding &c; and sups lightly on milk pottage &c; may with reason hope for health..
  'Let temperance constantly preside:
  Your best physician friend and guide'

Armstrong

The tone of *The Villager's Friend* is always one of friendliness until such time as a child's life is threatened. He has no qualms about highlighting the horrors of physical abuse:

> *This complaint (water on the brain) is frequently occasioned by the falls on the head, which children are exposed to on first going alone. Guard their heads… with the old fashioned head-dress for children… I am sorry to be obliged to add another cause of this malady, severe blows on the head, inflicted in the correction of children. Parents too often forget the weight of their hands, and the delicate structure of a child…. It was but yesterday I passed the cottage of one you all know to have always neglected his children; I hear the plaintive and suppliant cries of a child, and rushed into the cottage; where I saw the father, whose countenance was dreadful…beating most unmercifully his son, about ten years old. The poor child's countenance would, one would have supposed, obtained mercy from the most obdurate; it was shrunk up with dread and terror; the most earnest and humble supplications proceeded from his lips whilst his eyes were fixed with horror on the impending instrument of his chastisement. I stopped the brute from proceeding in his violent outrage asking what was the crime the boy had committed and found he had not completed the task of work he had set him…. The crimes of the children of such a parent must be on his head: you merit correction not he, for you never showed him what it was to be industrious. Expect not duty from a child if you have not done yours toward him…*

Parkinson also exhorts any doctor treating a child to approach the case with caution.

> *When this disease (erysipelas) appears on very young children, the loss of the child is only to be prevented by the most skilful exertions. Admit no tamperings, lest you have to accuse yourself of having thereby sacrificed the child of your heart…*

He also includes a scenario that would be familiar to many medical professionals in the twenty-first century:

> *Have you to consult your lawyer or to employ any other man almost in the village, you will require his attendance, at that time which may best suit his convenience; but should a trifling rash on the skin, which*

has hardly excited your attention for a week or two, at last induce you to call for the attendance of your apothecary, the application will frequently be deferred to the close of the day: nor will the roughest and most tempestuous weather excuse the attendance, which will, in general, be thought necessary to be insisted on directly, to give energy and effect to your message...

This writing continued well into the nineteenth century and in 1817 he published his *Essay on the Shaking Palsy*, which was to make his name. Little had been written about this disabling condition up until this time, and even then, many of the complaints made by Parkinson, most particularly of the inefficacy of treatments available to anyone suffering the distressing symptoms of the palsy are still relevant today: 'Involuntary tremulous motion, with lessened muscular power, in parts not in action and even when supported: with a propensity to bend the trunk forwards, and to pass from walking to a running pace: the senses and intellect being uninjured'. It did not make a widespread impression at the time, but later in the nineteenth century the French physician Jean-Martin Charcot read the paper and from there on it was referred to by him as 'maladie du Parkinson'. Progress in the treatment of Parkinson's has been very slow, however, and well into the twenty-first century the medical community still struggles to find long-term solutions to the difficulties patients face.

His expertise as a medical man was recognised by his peers, especially the Association of Apothecaries (of which he was elected president in 1817), who offered him the opportunity to be closely involved in the drafting and passing of the Apothecaries Act in 1815, which did so much to regulate the training of young surgeon-apothecaries and paved the way for the further development of an all-inclusive training for doctors.

It is also likely that the poet and fellow apothecary, John Keats (See Chapter 8) was familiar with Parkinson's paper, and there is much discussion about his use of the word 'palsy' in *Ode to a Nightingale* (Where palsy shakes a few, sad, last gray hairs) and *The Eve of St Agnes*, in which the old nurse, Angela, is 'palsy-stricken' and seen 'shuffling along'. In *The Fall of Hyperion*, Keats has Saturn calling his sickness a 'shaking palsy' and he exhibits that lack of muscular and vocal power so suggestive of the symptoms Parkinson describes.

James Parkinson died in December 1824 at the age of 69. He was much missed by the residents of Hoxton, who were then served by his son, also called James. The legacy of his decades of study of the effects of palsy lives on.

Thomas Paytherus – forgotten friend of Jenner?

There is not much to be found about Thomas Paytherus on the Internet. He does not have one of those ubiquitous Wikipedia entries that do at least point you in the way of some useful references. But research in the Wellcome Library and consultation of the *Journal of Medical Biography* led to the discovery of a piece written in 2013 by Henry Connor, a retired physician, and David M. Clark, a Historical Geographer. Called *Thomas Paytherus (1752-1828): Entrepreneurial surgeon-apothecary and ardent Jennerian*, the article gathers some interesting facts about a man who was not just a successful surgeon-apothecary, but a businessman and friend to Edward Jenner, pioneer of smallpox vaccination. How far his influence with, or support of, Jenner went is not clear, and there is little enough reference to Paytherus in books about Jenner's work, but in any event, Paytherus is a good example of the commercial spirit that helped many surgeon-apothecaries make a decent living in the late eighteenth and early nineteenth centuries.

Thomas Paytherus was born in 1752 in the village of Fownhope, which sits in the largely rural area east of Hereford. The industry in the countryside around the village is, as it was in Paytherus's time, agriculture, and Paytherus's father, Thomas Senior, was one in a long line of yeoman farmers who had lived in the village for more than 300 years. The family was comfortably off, owning a substantial amount of land, and at the age of 17, Thomas Junior was apprenticed to a surgeon at Gloucester Infirmary, at a premium of £200, a substantial sum at the time, but in line with premiums paid by other apprentices in that period.

As with many such arrangements, the agreement was made through personal contacts. The surgeon, Robert Browne Cheston, was the son of Joseph Cheston who owned land bordering that farmed by the Paytherus family in Fownhope, and he had, by the time he took young Paytherus on, already established himself at the infirmary and went on, in later years and after further qualification, to become Physician to the Infirmary. Thomas Paytherus would, therefore, have had a very capable teacher and the opportunity to study in an environment quite different from other men mentioned in this book. He was studying before the implementation of the Apothecaries Act 1815, which laid down a particular mode of study necessary to achieve the status of Licentiate of the Society of Apothecaries, but after his apprenticeship was completed, he furthered his medical education in London, studying under the radical young surgeon Henry Cline, a supporter of activists John Horne Tooke and John Thelwall, and of the French Revolution. As Connor and Clark point out, we know nothing of Thomas Paytherus's own political views, but Cline, subversive that he was, would not be the obvious choice of tutor in any event, being just two years older than his pupil, but he was to achieve high standing in the profession in later years and was, therefore, a very useful connection to have made.

Still, Paytherus sought to learn more, and moved to Edinburgh, probably in late 1775, to attend lectures in chemistry given by Joseph Black, an exceptional chemist and outstanding lecturer who filled the halls with students keen to hear him speak. Thomas does not appear to have attended with the intention of taking a degree, as he did not register as a student at the university and within eighteen months he was back in London where he qualified with the Diploma of the Royal Company of Surgeons in July 1777.

It is clear from this pattern of study that Paytherus was hoping to be something other than a small town or village general practitioner. He was, however, to be thwarted in any ambition he had to work as a surgeon at the hospital in which he had trained under Cheston, by the son of the man himself, Samuel Cheston, and there was no opening to be had at Hereford either, where posts were also held by one family for generations. So he moved to nearby Ross-on-Wye, with its developing tourist market, and entered into a partnership with local apothecary William Wood, who was by then already 77 years old. The businessman in Paytherus must have hoped his partner would soon take a genteel retirement, but again he was to be disappointed, as his senior partner enjoyed his work so much, and was himself so hale and hearty, that he continued working for more than a decade. Paytherus was, however, now in a position to take on his own apprentice, and received £170 to become a mentor to Richard Evans, who was later to become his partner.

So Thomas Paytherus took on the role many surgeon-apothecaries performed at that time and became a doctor to the poor of the local parish of Kings Caple, which, when the fees for midwifery and other services were added to the basic fee for care and medicine, boosted the doctor's income by around £10. When this sum is compared to the fees charged by medical men to their rich clients at the same period, the amount seems paltry, but Paytherus was not just interested in making money. It is clear from Connor and Clark's research that he was already interested in inoculation against smallpox and it is likely he encouraged the introduction of free inoculation into the parish in 1884.

In 1786, Thomas Paytherus was married to Frances Hodges, with whom he went on to have four children: a son and three daughters. He worked hard to establish his family in Ross-on-Wye and as soon as one apprentice had come to the end of his training he took on another, at an increased premium. Edward Jenner was later to suggest that his friend had worked so hard as 'surgeon and man-midwife' that he had damaged his own health.

Perhaps, then, it is not surprising that in 1794 he decided on a change of direction, and moved to London, where he established a 'Chemical, Drug and Medicinal Warehouse' and became a vigorous manufacturer, marketer and purveyor of proprietary medicines, with such names as 'The Chalybeate Aperient or true Cheltenham Salts', which purported to offer the purchaser the opportunity to dissolve them in water and enjoy the benefits of Cheltenham Spa without the expense of a visit to the town itself. Jenner was a great champion of the product and it was still being sold well into the nineteenth century. Alongside the salts, he sold preparations that were said to cure rickets, a nipple ointment to solve a problem nursing mothers were only too familiar with, and had the exclusive rights to make and sell Dr Jenner's Absorbent Digestive Lozenges.

Paytherus's business was a huge success and was patronised by the rich and famous, even dispensing prescriptions to the royal family. At this time Paytherus was also working as a surgeon-apothecary, taking on further apprentices at much higher premiums than he had been able to charge back in Ross-on-Wye, and his practice too saw patronage from a fashionable set. By this time he was a comparatively wealthy man, and working in partnership with Thomas Savory and Thomas Moore he built the business to the point that, when Savory and Moore (a company which continued trading until 1981) bought him out in 1811, they had to find around £25,000 to do so.

There is little doubt that Thomas Paytherus had always been an enthusiastic advocate of vaccination, despite the strong objections to the practice that were raised by influential doctors of the period. There is evidence to suggest that Buddhist monks drank snake venom to bestow an immunity to snake venom, and in the seventeenth century the Chinese used 'variolation', or the smearing of a cut in the skin with cowpox, to confer immunity to smallpox, but in the West it is Edward Jenner, long-time friend of Paytherus, who is credited with the founding of widespread vaccinology in its modern form. He was certainly the man who was prepared to work hard to establish the procedure and push for a widespread vaccination programme, despite years struggling to convince the medical hierarchy that such a commitment could save countless lives. Jenner was ridiculed and many, especially many clergymen, claimed it was 'ungodly' to use matter from a diseased animal to inoculate a human being. A cartoon of 1802 shows people given Jenner's vaccination growing a cow's head, and the government seemed unable to make a decision on how best to proceed. Throughout those years, correspondence shows Thomas Paytherus to be one of Jenner's staunchest supporters, who was present at meetings where Jenner sought the advice of his peers on how best to proceed and, during a particularly bitter exchange with a Dutch doctor, Jan Ingen Housz, it is clear Jenner had such faith in his friend that he appointed him to act as intermediary between the two men, although it seems there was no convincing Dr Ingen Hausz of the merits of Jenner's claims.

In subsequent years, Thomas Paytherus was also to alert Edward Jenner to the work of another doctor in the field, thus ensuring Jenner was prepared to publish the findings of his research before others had the opportunity to take the credit. As an important member of the Royal Jennarian Society, Paytherus was always prepared to defend Jenner against claims that the vaccination was unsafe, or that it failed to provide the protection Jenner claimed, and regularly acted as Jenner's agent in London.

In their paper, Connor and Clark quote from a letter written by Jenner to Thomas Paytherus in 1808, when Jenner was clearly frustrated with the difficulties he continued to face:

> *Vaccination will go on just as well when I am dead as it does during my existence, probably better, for one obstacle will die with me – Envy.... If I could obtain a little peace and quietness, my pockets should readily restore every shilling they have gained by the cow-pox discovery. That such a thing has been discovered, I, with the rest of mankind have reason to rejoice; but this I also declare, that I wish it had been the lot of some other person to have been the discoverer...*

Connor and Clark's research suggests that Paytherus retired from active medical practice when he moved out of London around 1810 and that he enjoyed a lengthy retirement, working on his gardens and moving in and out of the capital until 1828, when he died at his family home in Abergavenny on 5 June at the age of 76. His family had remained close to the Jenner family, but his friend Edward had died five years previously, on 26 January 1823. Paytherus's death was largely unremarked upon in the press, either local or medical. His wife died two years later, and the family was left well provided for. None of their three daughters married, and their son seems to have married but died without issue.

Thomas Paytherus worked hard; from his relatively quiet beginnings as a surgeon-apothecary and general practitioner in the Herefordshire countryside, he became a man of some means in the fashionable circles in London and played no small part in supporting a friend who is today recognised as one of the great medical men of the age.

Chapter 8

Three men of Guy's – Keats, Stephens and Thackrah

From pills to poetry – John Keats

It is a better and a wiser thing to be a starved apothecary than a starved poet; so back to the shop, Mr John, back to the 'plaster, pills and ointment boxes &c. But for Heaven's sake, Young Sangrado, be a little more sparing of extenuatives and soporifics in your practice than you have been in your poetry

When John Gibson Lockhart of *Blackwood's Edinburgh Review* wrote this stinging review of John Keats's *Endymion* in 1818, he could little have imagined the long-term impact it would have on Keats's reputation. The poet himself was hurt, but not mortally so, as many of his friends and contemporaries would say after his death from tuberculosis in 1821, at the age of just 25. He was, until his illness, a strong, stocky young man, passionate and with an occasionally fiery temper, interested in the real world and the radical politics of the day.

For decades after his death, Keats was depicted as a frail youth, disillusioned by the attacks and driven to an early grave. His friends perpetuated this image to a certain extent and fellow Romantic poet Percy Bysshe Shelley wrote a whole poem dedicated to him, called *Adonais,* in which he loudly declared his belief that the reviews had contributed to his death.

Far from Lockwood's jibe that Keats was simply a pretty boy practising 'poetry and pharmacy'; it is now known how important medical training was to Keats and his development as a poet, and of his personal and poetical philosophy. Keats's fame has also contributed to the scholarship devoted to the lives of students of medicine at the time, as authors determine to examine the minute details of his life in order to find influences in his work. Biographies have discovered much about his training at Guy's Hospital in London, if not about the years spent as an apprentice in Edmonton, then a village to the north of London.

John Keats was born on or around 31 of October 1795 and baptised in December at St Botolph's Church, Bishopsgate. His exact birthplace is unknown but at that time his father, Thomas Keats, and mother, Frances Keats née Jennings, were living in Moorgate on the edge of the City of London.

Keats was raised in Moorfields, on London Wall. His father and mother ran 'The Swan and Hoop' and livery stables, close to the notorious Bethlem Lunatic Asylum, better known as 'Bedlam'.

In April 1804 his father had a serious riding accident on his way home from visiting his sons at school. He was rendered insensible by a fall and died the following day. To add to this trauma, his mother seemed to disappear from the children's lives, only to return just weeks later, re-married to William Rawlings, and from that period onwards the boys had to spend school holidays with their grandparents.

1809 saw the celebrated the return of his mother to the Jennings household, but she was a sick woman and was only to live a further year, dying in March 1810.

The artist Benjamin Robert Haydon wrote later, in his diary: 'Before his mother died, during her last illness, his devoted attachment interested all. He sat up whole nights in a great chair, would suffer nobody to give her medicine but himself, and even cooked her food; he did all, & read novels in her intervals of ease.' Her loss may have been the inspiration for his medical career.

It is impossible to know for certain whether to enter into the apprenticeship with Hammond was his own idea or not. Charles Cowden Clarke suggests it was not, as did Joseph Severn, the artist and friend of Keats, who nursed him during his final illness in Rome. However, there was a tradition of medical training in the Keats family, and Nicholas Roe, in his 2012 biography of the poet, suggests that the apprenticeship was presented by Keats's legal guardian, Richard Abbey, as a 'fait accompli', but one which was not altogether against Keats's will. The Keats family was not wealthy, but the inheritance left to John, George, Tom and Fanny by parents and grandparents would offer enough to establish the boys in respectable trades.

As we have seen in Chapter 1, an apothecary was not viewed as having a high social status in the early nineteenth century, but the role would hopefully provide a secure income. John Keats was apprenticed to the Keats and Jennings family doctor, Thomas Hammond. As with many similar apprenticeships, this was a private arrangement and did not involve the Society of Apothecaries. Hammond had a good reputation and came from a family of medical men. He had trained at Guy's and St Thomas's hospitals, in London, which would offer John Keats the advantage of connections when he followed his master to the same hospitals after his apprenticeship ended.

Keats and one other apprentice lived above the brick built surgery and dispensary in the grounds of the house, which was typical of many another apothecaries' premises. A ground floor room was panelled with wood and shelving on a dresser, where Hammond prepared and stored his medicinal preparations.

Thomas Hammond charged £200 for Keats to be bound as his apprentice, covering his board and education. Hammond would have promised 'meat, drink and lodging' and 'proper physic & other necessaries', should Keats fall ill. For his part, the 15-year-old Keats promised to live a life away from taverns and gambling dens.

The biographies of the other men in this book suggest regular tasks included cleaning and dusting, sorting bottles, filling some with leeches, and rolling pills, which could become mundane if the master did not offer the apprentice interesting new tasks to develop their skills and give them the chance to take greater responsibility. Keats resented tasks such as sweeping floorboards and holding Hammond's horse, waiting whilst his master went into a house to treat a patient.

Over time Keats could watch and learn as Hammond dressed wounds, removed teeth, and diagnosed minor complaints such as constipation. Knowledge of more serious illness and the chance to treat it would have come in time and as Roe states, Keats may have seen 'fractures, dislocations, gunshot wounds, intestinal obstructions, tapeworms, burns and scalds, difficult births, congenital malformations, tumours, convulsions, gout, accidents, diseases, hernias and so on'.

Hammond would have set fractures, amputated limbs, removed bladder stones and attempted to repair harelips – all 'minor' conditions that could be attempted with success at this time. Of course, each procedure would have been undertaken without anaesthetic. A well-trained apothecary would, especially after the 1815 Apothecaries Act required them to gain experience in surgery on the wards of teaching hospitals, be more skilled with patients and have a greater knowledge of general medicine and minor surgery than more specialised physicians trained solely at the university medical schools.

Eventually, Keats vented his frustration at his treatment and, as he described years later in a letter to his brother George and sister-in-law Georgiana, his 'hand clench'd itself' against Hammond. We have no further details of that occasion, but despite the many studies and biographies that assume Keats completed the full five years of his apprenticeship, the consensus is now that it is unlikely that it went to full term. According to an earlier biographer, Sidney Colvin, a fellow apprentice of Hammond described Keats as 'an idle loafing fellow, always writing poetry', although none of that work has survived.

In any event, if Keats's apprenticeship did not run its course, there must have been an alternative medical education available to him, as he was fully prepared and qualified to enrol as a student at Guy's Hospital in 1815. His dislike of Hammond had clearly not put him off the eventual practice of medicine.

Nicholas Roe has put forward the possibility that the gap between the early ending of his apprenticeship and the beginning of his training in London may have been filled with voluntary attendance at lectures held regularly at St Thomas's and Guy's Hospitals. The history of Charles Turner Thackrah's medical training (see later in this chapter) makes this more likely; Thackrah was an exact contemporary of Keats and was a keen attendee of these lectures.

Hammond did return Keats's indenture documents. These documents were possessed by apprentices in all trades and bound them to their apprenticeship, and Keats would, on enrolment at Guy's, still fulfil all the necessary entry requirements.

There has always been a certain mystery about the speed with which Keats seemed to rise to prominence at Guy's Hospital. Sir Astley Cooper himself appeared to take more than an ordinary interest in his career, helping him to find his lodging close to the hospital, at 28 St Thomas Street in Southwark, or the 'Borough'. In 1815 this was a notoriously squalid area; streets of dilapidated timbered tenements, open ditches full of foul waste, and prostitutes and thieves were commonplace in what Keats described as 'a beastly place in dirt, turnings and windings'. Situated as it was at the southern end of London Bridge, along the main road into Kent, the roads were jammed with coaches and waggon loads of provisions making their way in and out of the City.

Keats's landlord was a tallow chandler called Markham who rented out study bedrooms and a communal sitting room to students. John first shared with two much older and more senior students, Frederick Tyrrell and George Cooper, but when they had finished their studies Keats asked George Wilson Mackereth and Henry Stephens to share his rooms to cover the £63 per year rent, a sum well above his sole means.

On Sunday 1 October 1815, John Keats registered at Guy's Hospital in London. He would have signed the necessary paperwork in the Counting House, handing over the fee of £1 2s to cover a twelve-month period. The next day he registered as a surgical pupil for the same period, at the cost of £25 4s.

It seems Keats was a successful student. He didn't miss lectures, attended classes in dissection, and passed his examinations to become a member of the Society of Apothecaries when many others, including Henry Stephens, failed the first time. As well as the assistance with housing, within months Keats took on the role of dresser over candidates who had been at the hospital for much longer. This suggests a real ambition to become a surgeon, as a dressership was seen as far superior to the education gained by becoming a 'mere pupil' (Aesculapius). But R.S. White, in his article *'Esculapius of Old' – Keats Medical Training*, thinks that it might be during the second six months of this training that he may have re-read his *Hospital Pupil* again and realised that as a surgeon he could not be 'deaf to the pains of his patient' to obtain a 'lasting good' and that his healing powers were best expressed by use of a pen rather than a scalpel.

The position of dresser was something of an honour for a student, particularly those from less wealthy backgrounds. As a surgical pupil, a man would have been expected to 'walk the wards', observe the surgeons and ask pertinent questions. Those with money could pay hundreds of pounds to become a surgeon's apprentice, with the attendant additional opportunities to ask questions and gain experience. To be offered the position of 'dresser', a role between that of pupil and apprentice, meant that the student gained a few additional privileges, but rather more responsibility. Each surgeon could have up to four dressers, which meant that at Guy's there were just twelve young men, each of whom had to live in for a week at a time, on a rota. A bedroom and sitting room were provided, but the dresser had to meet the expense from his own pocket.

John Flint South described in detail the duties of a dresser:

> *He attended to all the accidents and cases of a hernia which came in during his week in office, and he dressed hosts of out-patients, drew innumerable teeth, and performed countless venesections, till two or three o'clock, as might be, till the surgery was emptied.... When the surgeon arrived the dresser on duty would show him, among the outpatients, any case about which he needed further help or which he thought advisable to be admitted, as likely to issue in an operation.... Cases of strangulated hernia, retention of urine, and other accidents, were admitted at the discretion of the dresser.*

The dresser would carry a 'plaster box', from which he would take plasters and bandages to dress the patients' wounds as instructed by his surgeon, and he would also administer any drugs prescribed. The dresser would also be responsible for calling a surgeon should an emergency arise, and at night they might be responsible for dealing with these major cases themselves.

The most relevant period for the purposes of this book is the period between his enrolment at Guy's Hospital in 1815, and the spring of 1817, when we can with confidence say Keats had given up his medical studies for literary ones. During his short life post-Guy's (he left aged 21 and died aged 25) he mentioned returning to a medical career in his letters to friends, and had kept his medical textbooks, but there is no doubt that had he returned to practice as a doctor it would have been from economic necessity rather than vocation.

Keats moved to London to study medicine at a critical time for both apothecaries and surgeons. In Chapter 1 the ways in which the structure of the medical profession changed are given in more detail, but at this point it is useful to remember that although the passing of the Apothecaries Act in 1815 laid down firm requirements for students intending to qualify for membership of the Society of Apothecaries, at the same time the College of Surgeons was in a state of flux. Established just fifteen years before the Apothecaries Act, it did not yet have a building to act as a focal point for governance or licensing and didn't get the royal charter until 1822. Only then did it have any power to regulate the profession and had less rigorous requirements than the London Society of Apothecaries. Only two years before Keats enrolled at Guy's there was a formal recognition of the need for a practising surgeon to have, at the very least, a certificate proving surgical attendance at a hospital. When Keats was studying, neither the Society of Apothecaries nor the College of Surgeons was a teaching institution, and men with a variety of backgrounds, studied at the larger hospitals and at private anatomy schools, and simply sat for the qualifying examinations.

Astley Cooper gave lectures on 'The Principles and Practice of Surgery' in the evenings from October 1815 (when Keats enrolled) to 1 June 1816, and 'Anatomy and the Principal Operations of Surgery' in the first half of 1816. We know Keats at least started this course, as his medical notebook from this period has survived.

Cooper was a pupil of John Hunter, revolutionary anatomist, whose vast collection of anatomical specimens form the centrepiece of the Hunterian Museum in London. Cooper's style and flamboyant nature attracted students to him and his appearance in the lecture hall would immediately cast a spell over the audience. John Flint South described him:

A few moments before two Astley Cooper came briskly through the crowd, his handsome face beaming with delight and animation. He was dressed in black, with short knee breeches and silk stockings, which well-displayed his handsome legs, of which he was not a little proud. Almost to a minute he was in the theatre, where loud and continued greetings most truly declared the affectionate regard his pupils had for him. His clear, silvery voice and cheery conversational manner soon exhausted the conventional hour devoted to the lecture; and all who heard him hung with silent attention on his words, the only sounds which broke the quiet being the subdued pen-scratching of the note takers...

Astley Cooper was 'implicitly trusted'. He was also known for the generosity with which he shared his medical discoveries. It is likely that all the medical men covered in this book would have been taught by, or at least have come into contact with the writings of, the great man. He was made a Baronet in 1821, having successfully treated the King, and was known as the 'outstanding British surgeon of his time'.

Up to 400 students would attend his lectures at one time, and Keats, like many of his contemporaries, would have been in thrall to the great man. Apart from the direct evidence of his notebook, Astley Cooper's ideas and philosophy of medicine can be directly traced through Keats's own development of a philosophy of poetry.

John Barnard points out that, owing to his early appointment as a dresser, when Keats passed his apothecary's examinations he needed just a further two months hospital experience to meet the requirements of the College of Surgeons. Knowing as we do that he continued his role as a dresser, probably until the spring of 1817, his abandonment of medicine for poetry came at the point when he could have qualified as a fully-fledged surgeon-apothecary, as both Waddington and Thackrah went on to do.

This might go some way to explain the response of his legal guardian, Richard Abbey when Keats told him of his decision to pursue a career in poetry, rather than set up in practice close to his boyhood home in Edmonton:

[Abbey] *communicated his plans to his Ward, but his Surprise was not moderate, to hear in Reply, that he did not intend to be a Surgeon – Not intend to be a Surgeon! Why what do you mean to be? I mean to rely on my Abilities as a Poet – John, you are either mad or a Fool, to talk in so absurd a Manner. My mind is made up said the youngster very quietly. I know that I possess Abilities greater than most Men, and therefore I am determined to gain my Living by exercising them. – Seeing nothing could be done Abby* [sic] *...called...him a Silly Boy. & prophesied a speedy Termination to his inconsiderate Enterprise.*

Andrew Motion in *Keats*

Keats had made a success of his training, and he had completed it, but his mind was indeed made up.

Donald C. Goellnicht in *The Poet-Physician – Keats and Medical Science*, has also made a study of the training young men like Keats undertook in this period. The United Hospitals of Guy's and St Thomas's were well respected and the medical training offered was far from perfunctory or ad hoc. The course offered in the autumn term included 'Anatomy and the operations of Surgery', by Mr Astley Cooper and Mr Henry Cline at St Thomas's, and at Guy's Hospital, the 'Practice of Medicine', 'Experimental Philosophy', 'Theory of Medicine and Materia Medica' and 'Diseases of Women and children' were taught by Drs Babington, Curry Marcet, Haighton and Cholmley, along with Mr Allen and Mr Fox.

The timetable was established so as to avoid clashes and ensure students could complete 'a complete course of medical and chirurgical instruction'.

After the implementation of the Apothecaries Act in 1815, Guy's Hospital was also able to offer courses in anatomy and surgery, as well as those in medicine, making it the hospital of choice for those seeking the all-round education necessary for a surgeon-apothecary.

As well as the courses of Cooper and Cline, Keats is known to have signed up for two courses on the Practice of Medicine, taught by Drs Babington and Curry, two on Chemistry by Drs Babington, Marcet and Mr Allen, and one on the Theory of Medicine and Materia Medica taught by Drs Curry and Cholmley. Nicholas Roe suggests that '...he almost certainly attended Astley Cooper's evening lectures on 'Principles and Practice of Surgery', which began at 8pm on the Monday, just a week after his enrolment. These lectures were of use to Keats mainly as a future surgeon, reinforcing the probability that he intended to obtain the qualifications necessary to work as surgeon-apothecary.

John Flint South, as well as describing the charismatic Cooper, was an acute observer if the peculiarities of other lecturers. Babington would attend, still dirty and reeking of the dissecting room, but clear and practical. Curry 'performed in a haze of powder, wearing a silver sand-wig, extravagant shirt and neck cloth, gold watch and a chunky ring on his little finger'.

Despite the inspirational lectures, Astley Cooper made it clear to students that 'anatomical knowledge cannot be perfect unless [the student] has frequently seen and assisted in the dissection of the human body'. Whatever the student's finer feelings they must be put aside, according to the surgeon in charge of the dissecting room in Keats's time, demonstrator of anatomy, surgeon Joseph Henry Green:

> *It is not sufficient that he is merely acquainted with the presence of certain parts, but he must know precisely their situation and extent. The surgeon's knife may give health or death within the space of a hair's breadth. This kind of knowledge is to be acquired by actual dissection alone.*

In *Life of Keats*, Charles Brown gives the reason for his great friend Keats leaving medicine as not simply the need to pursue a career as a poet, but a genuine fear of making that slip, a 'hair's breadth between life and death'.

> *He ascribed his inability to an overwrought apprehension of every possible chance of doing evil in the wrong direction of the instrument. 'My last operation,' he told me 'was the opening of a man's temporal artery. I did it with the utmost nicety; but, reflecting on what passed through my mind at the time, my dexterity seemed a miracle, and I never took up the lancet again.'*

This is hardly surprising bearing in mind his experience in surgery. When Keats was offered the role of 'dresser' on 29 October 1815, to start the following March, he had been a student for less than a month. It is possible that attendance at lectures after his apprenticeship ended early – but before signing up as a student – had already brought him to the attention of Cooper and Cline and highlighted his potential, but as he was only just on the cusp of 20 years old; this was a rapid promotion. He was not assigned to Cooper, however, but to William Lucas Junior, the son of Thomas Hammond's master at Guy's. South described Lucas as:

> *A tall, ungainly awkward man, with stooping shoulders and shuffling walk, as deaf as a post, not overburdened with brains of any kind, but very good-natured and easy, and liked by everyone. His surgical acquirements were very small, his operations generally very badly performed, and accompanied with much bungling, if not worse. He was a poor anatomist and not a very good diagnose, which now and then led him into ugly scrapes.*

Astley Cooper broke protocol to agree that Lucas was: 'neat-handed but rash in the extreme, cutting amongst most important parts as though they were only skin, and making us all shudder from the apprehension of his opening arteries or committing some other horror'.

In the early nineteenth century, operations were rushed affairs, for speed was vital to stem the copious bleeding and prevent the patient, lying restrained on the wooden table at the centre of the operating theatre, dying of shock, as there was at the time no proper anaesthesia. The semi-circular operating theatres at Guy's and St Thomas's were too small to cope with the crush of students keen to get a glimpse of a great surgeon at work.

Following the operation, it was left to the dresser to dress the wound and he would continue to do so daily in order to prevent, as far as was possible, infection setting in.

It is not known for certain why Keats gave up medicine in 1817, although it was obviously not because he did not have the constitution or application for it. The anecdotes of contemporary and housemate Henry Stephens (see later in this chapter) suggest that Keats never fully engaged with his studies, and thought himself rather above them:

> *It may readily be imagined that this feeling was accompanied with a good deal of Pride and some conceit, and that amongst mere Medical students, he would walk, & talk as one of the Gods might be supposed to do, when mingling with mortals. This pride had exposed him, as may be readily imagined, to occasional ridicule, & some mortification.*

It is clear from Stephens's accounts that there was a certain amount of jealousy of Keats's rise to prominence at the hospital, and his ability to pass, with ease, an exam that Stephens had failed at the first time of asking.

Rather than a lack of application to his studies, Keats was quick to learn and Brown's quote rather suggests that Keats felt he could not maintain the control necessary to hold the clear focus Astley Cooper maintained was necessary for a good surgeon: 'But the quality which is considered of the highest order in surgical operations is self-possession; the head must always direct the hand, otherwise the operator is unfit to discover and effectual remedy for the unforeseen accidents which may occur in his practice.'

Far from being too sensitive to the horrors of early nineteenth century medical treatments and the sights and smells of the hospital ward, it seems Keats took Cooper's warnings about the importance of a single-minded and dedicated devotion to surgical duty to heart, and considered that his fear of failure, allied with his increasing interest in a career in poetry, to exclude him from surgery as a career.

Doctor, chemist, inventor – Henry Stephens

Henry Stephens was born in 1796, in Holborn London, but within two years his father, Joseph, and mother, Catherine, moved Henry and his elder brother, John, out of the densely populated capital to the rural county of Hertfordshire. After the birth of Henry's two younger siblings, sisters Frances and Catherine, the family settled in Redbourn, a village north of St Albans where another son was born: Samuel Josiah.

The village of Redbourn is on the famous 'Watling Street', the Roman road that became the major coaching route between London and the north-west of England, and the Stephens family took charge of the main inn on the High Street. The Bull was a stop on the route of many a traveller's journey, offering the opportunity for refreshment and a change of horses for the hundred or more coaches that travelled that way each day (and night).

Henry developed a lifetime's love of horses but did not want to follow in his parents' footsteps. He wanted to be a doctor, and despite Redbourn's lack of medical facilities at that period, he was able to find an apprenticeship in a neighbouring village. Markyate, approximately three miles from Redbourn, was home to surgeon John Winkfield, and apothecary Benjamin Somers, who agreed to take Henry on as an apprentice at the age of about 14. He was happy there for the five years of his training, lodging with Winkfield and his wife in their substantial home in the village.

It seems his life as an apprentice followed the usual pattern. In the earliest stages, he would have accompanied Winkfield on his rounds, helping with dressings as required. By the end of his apprenticeship, his skills would have increased to the point where he could make a sound diagnosis of common ailments, dress wounds and treat fractures, prescribe suitable medications and even deliver babies.

The end of Stephens's apprenticeship coincided with the implementation of the Apothecaries Act 1815, which required all those aspiring to set up in practice to complete an approved course of lectures, work on the wards of a teaching hospital for six months, and pass two, not insignificant, examinations set by both the Society of Apothecaries and Royal College of Surgeons. This increased the cost of becoming a doctor considerably; although we do not know exactly how much Stephens paid for his studies, the £1,500 it cost to train John Keats in the same period equates to something over £60,000 in the twenty-first century.

Henry Stephens was clearly in possession of the necessary funds, as he made the decision to enrol in one of the most forward thinking and dynamic of the teaching hospitals, the United Hospitals of Guy's and St Thomas's in Southwark, (see Chapter 2). On 14 October 1815 he paid his £1 2s fee to cover his formal enrolment, and two days later, paid a further eighteen guineas to attend the wards for a period of six months, increasing by a further six guineas in November when he realised he had misunderstood the period necessary to qualify as both Licentiate of the Society of Apothecaries (LSA) and Member of the Royal College of Surgeons (MRCS). A further fee was due to attend the compulsory lectures and other formal instruction.

From the leafy lanes of Hertfordshire to the streets of central London was a mere thirty-five miles by coach from his home, but it was a world away from the streets in which Stephens now had to find lodgings. The filth of the streets and the poverty of the residents of this overcrowded area were impossible to ignore, but there is no evidence to suggest that Stephens was unhappy there. The lodgings he found at 28 St Thomas Street were close to the hospital, although not cheap. Robert Gittings, in his biography of John Keats, with whom Stephen's eventually shared a sitting room, states that the cost per resident was approximately £63 per annum, reduced on the sharing of the sitting room with another. In the first instance, Henry shared with George Mackereth, who had also recently enrolled following an apprenticeship in Lincolnshire, but after only two months or so, Keats was left alone in the lodgings he had shared in the same building, and asked Stephens and Mackareth if he could reduce his outgoings by sharing their sitting room. The agreement lasted around one year and sealed Stephen's place in literary history as one of the only direct witnesses to this period of the great poet's life.

His reminiscences for Victorian biographies of Keats are not wholly reliable; Stephens was rather sour about Keats's early promotion to dresser at Guy's and felt that the poet's success was largely due to good Latin rather than good medical knowledge. The men also disagreed on matters poetical (Stephens has his own literary ambition and was possibly envious of Keats's success as a poet, and Keats for his part struck Stephens as proud). However, their friendship was sufficiently sound for them to meet after their training was over; for example, Keats visited Stephens in Redbourn in 1818 just before his walking trip to the North and Scotland.

Henry Stephens's training took the familiar pattern. He would have attended the lectures in the two terms from October to January, and then from late January until mid-May, with formal instruction suspended for the hottest of the summer months. This was not to offer the students any kind of leisure time, however, it was a necessity at a time when dead bodies for use in anatomy and dissection were in short supply and the 'specimens' horrific enough even when the weather was cold.

Full details of the lecture courses and other instruction Henry Stephens would have undertaken are given in an earlier chapter, but they included the aforementioned Anatomy and Physiology, the Theory and Practice of Medicine and Chemistry (a subject that Stephen's would pursue until his death) and Materia Medica.

In the summer of 1816, all three students took the examination to be accepted as an LSA. Only one passed – Keats. Stephens and Mackareth had to wait almost a year to pass and be accepted, although they had, unlike Keats (who had ended his studies to become a full-time poet), taken and passed their examination in surgery, becoming MRCS, in the meantime. Henry Stephens and George Mackareth remained friends for life, and on 28 April 1863, his eldest son Henry married Margaret, George Mackareth's daughter.

Henry Stephens was now a qualified surgeon-apothecary and decided to practice back in his home village, which had only recently had its own 'poor doctor' appointed by the vestry. He is believed to have lived in a house opposite The Bull Inn, still run by his parents, and he was popular with patients from all social classes. In Chapter 5, this book looked in detail at the types of medical issues he would have been faced with in a rural practice, and at the treatments available to him at the time. There is little doubt that, like his contemporaries in other parts of the country, he would have seen some very distressing sights and been frustrated at the lack of effective treatments with which to counter the problems faced by poor and wealthy alike.

He was a paid doctor to the poor from 1820 and also vet to the hounds on a nearby estate, his treatment of one dog there being mentioned in his most notable published work of the period, a treatise on 'Hernia and the Mechanical Obstructions of the Bowels Internally', first published in 1829. He was encouraged by the great surgeon (and his former lecturer at Guy's) Astley Cooper to leave his home village at about this time and take his chances back in London, returning to Southwark and taking a large house close to the great hospitals. His treatise went into a second edition and although criticised by some, it was generally well received and his practice was successful. He also became a member of the Council of the Medical Society London, attending regular meetings and taking the opportunity to talk about his expertise in the treatment of a hernia, although its reception was apparently lukewarm in that instance, but he continued to attend, and was regularly elected to, the Council, which was responsible for the administration of the society.

However, during this time he also experienced tragedy, as he was to lose both his young wife and toddler daughter to consumption, and he had to continue his exhausting work with an even heavier workload during the outbreak of cholera that began in 1831, a disease that he took a significant interest in, particularly when he diagnosed himself with it in 1832, shortly after the death of his wife. His unlikely survival meant that his diagnosis was felt by some to be suspect, but there were instances of resistance noted by other doctors and he may only have suffered a mild dose.

Evidence suggests that it is soon after this difficult time that Stephens's interests moved away from becoming an expert in matters medical, although he continued to be a well-respected doctor in London, even when he removed his family to the more genteel and (then) rural area of Finchley, just a few miles from the city. Stephens is now best known for his invention of Stephens' Ink, which may have been prompted by the proximity of his home in Southwark to the Clowes printing works, and was certainly influenced by his dislike of the only available writing inks at that time. In 1838, an advertisement in Robson's London Directory offers 'Stephens's Patent Writing Fluids' in Carbonaceous Black, Dark Blue, Light Blue and Brilliant Red, sold in bottles at sixpence, a shilling and three shillings each, by 'Stationers and Booksellers'.

His indelible blue-black ink was exhibited at the Great Exhibition of 1851 and his company was soon producing great quantities of the ink, along with a number of other stationery items. Stephens's development of an indigo ink might not have been original, but he was a part of a group of entrepreneurial chemists (a subject supported by his medical training) who took the idea forward and was the most commercially successful. Stephens' Ink continued in production until the 1960s when the company was taken over; the ink remained in the company name until the mid-eighties.

Sadly, Henry Stephens died suddenly in 1864, and his medical career was not taken up by any members of his family. He had married for a second time, to Anne O'Reilly, in 1840 and had five children, the eldest of whom, Henry Charles, took on the mantle of head of the ink production company.

It is arguable, however, that it was during his medical career that Stephens made the most direct impact on people's lives, as he took his training and interest in chemistry and biology on to benefit the residents of Southwark and Finchley. The young student, known best now as the inventor of a famous ink brand and a sometime friend of the poet John Keats, had been a general practitioner to poor and wealthy alike and was deeply mourned by his friends, including scientist Michael Faraday.

Charles Turner Thackrah – the father of occupational medicine

Charles Turner Thackrah died at the age of just 38, but in his short life acquired a reputation that has ensured he is remembered both as a pioneer of occupational medicine and as a co-founder of the Leeds School of Medicine, where his name still graces the Institute of Health Sciences, and where a series of lectures is named after him. Short biographies were prepared after his death, but it was not until the 1950s that a more comprehensive essay on his work was written by A. Meiklejohn and attached to the work that made Thackrah's name – *The Effects of Arts, Trades and Professions and of civic states and habits of living on Health and Longevity: with suggestions for removal of many of the agents which produce disease and shorten the duration of life*, published in 1831.

Charles Turner Thackrah was born in Leeds on 22 May 1795 and baptised in St John's Church Briggate on 13 July. His father, George Thackrah, was a chemist and druggist in Leeds, but his mother, Alice, was keen that her son should follow her successful brother, the Reverend John Leader, into the church. Consequently, Charles was sent to study first with the Reverend Thomas Harrison of Bardsey, close to Leeds, and then to the Reverend Hammond Robertson, who ran a boarding school at Healds Hall, in Liversedge in the present-day borough of Kirklees. Robertson was a man staunchly to the right in politics and fiercely opposed to the Luddites. He was a significant enough character in the area to influence the work of Charlotte Bronte, who modelled her vicar, the Reverend Helstone in *Shirley*, on him. Apparently stern and merciless, and lacking in warmth, he was also known as a man of courage, albeit a controversial one.

Charles then moved on to Halifax, to be taught Divinity by the Reverend James Knight; by all accounts, including his own later writings, these men were good teachers who inspired in him a lifelong love of the Classics and of English Literature, subjects he would later encourage his own medical apprentices to read widely in. At the age of just 26 he was chosen to deliver a 'discourse' to the Leeds Philosophical and Literary Society in which he states:

> *But the pleasure which classical Learning confers, and the excitement which it affords, are not its only advantages. It also teaches the student to reason and to write. While it calls into action the intellectual energies, it imparts fluency of diction, and copiousness of illustration.*

Despite his early education and the encouragement of his mother, it was to his father's occupation that Charles was attracted. When he was 16, in 1811, he was apprenticed to a well-known Leeds surgeon and apothecary, Obadiah Brooke, for a period of five years, and was lucky enough to spend the final year of that apprenticeship attending as a pupil at Leeds Infirmary, just after the famous surgeon William Hey had retired and his son, also William, was making his name.

Like Keats and Stephens, Charles Turner Thackrah ended his apprenticeship at a time when training as a doctor was changing significantly, with the enactment of The Apothecaries Act 1815. After leaving Obadiah Brooke, he was required to attend a hospital, gain experience on the wards and attend a series of lectures in medicine and the medical sciences, and like Keats was also attracted to Guy's Hospital in London. Guy's was known at the time as the hospital around which all the most famous names and greatest innovators in medicine were congregating, and with its sister hospital, St Thomas's, it provided a combined surgical and medical education that was ahead of the other schools at the time.

In 1816, changes were also made to the profession of surgery, which required thenceforth that all surgeons wishing to practice had to be admitted as a member of the Royal College of Surgeons. The young men training at the time were privileged to be instructed in surgery by Astley Cooper who was a significant influence on Thackrah's later life and career, to the point where, Meiklejohn suggests, he even copied 'his somewhat flamboyant and oftentimes theatrical mode of presentation'.

Thackrah was an enthusiastic young man who threw himself into his studies, taking every opportunity to undertake extra-curricular activities, such as membership of the Physical Society, at which he presented his inaugural paper just a few weeks after taking up his place at the school, and was later to win a prize for his essay on diabetes.

There are a number of parallels between Thackrah's life and that of John Keats, not only their contemporaneous study at Guy's. Whilst he was still studying, Thackrah was taken ill with what were, for him, apparently episodic attacks of pain and diarrhoea that would affect him for the rest of his life. It is possible that this was an early indicator of the chronic pulmonary tuberculosis that was to kill him at the age of 38. John Keats died of the same disease aged 25, and it was reported to be an illness common amongst pupils subjected to the horrors of the dissecting room.

Thackrah passed all the examinations of the Royal College of Surgeons and of the Society of Apothecaries aged just 20, despite the fact that the

Society of Apothecaries required him to be 21. It is indicative of his general demeanour of the time; he was simply not prepared to wait for mandatory age requirements, and ultimately the Society, knowing he had reached the required standard, waved him through.

Thackrah decided to return to Leeds, but he was not a well man and, as Meiklejohn discovered, first exhibited signs of a melancholic nature that was at odds with his usual enthusiastic approach to life. These mood swings and changes in temperament might also have been a sign of incipient tuberculosis. He wrote in a letter to a friend: 'On a temperament like mine, naturally melancholic, with feelings naturally keen – at times, alas! Painfully acute – the common trials and disappointments of life produce an effect which is unknown to a man of less sensibility.'

He must have been under considerable strain, but the reason for it is not clear. He may always have been prone to melancholy, and have chosen to exhaust himself with work and study in order to distract himself from a low mood.

In 1817 Thackrah tried to establish a practice of his own, but as we have seen, it was not always easy for a man to gain success locally and despite his good medical education he would have experienced resistance from general practitioners of medicine already working in the city. However, that same year he was appointed 'town surgeon', which was not so grand a role as it sounds, offering little influence at local hospitals and poor payment, the role's main responsibility being the treatment of Poor Law patients in the worst slums in Leeds.

Keen to continue his studies and research, and increasingly respected in the local area as a doctor, and as a speaker, he was frustrated by his own poor health, and Meiklejohn makes an interesting comparison, once again, between Keats and Thackrah. At around this time – 1821 – Keats lost his own battle against tuberculosis, after spending the winter months in Rome with his friend Joseph Severn in a final attempt to ease the progression of the disease. At this time, Thackrah was also chronically ill and, once again it seems, in a low mood. After a very successful address to the Philosophical and Literary Society and at his most theatrical and melodramatic, he wrote:

I fear I shall be obliged to leave my native place and settle in some distant town; perhaps my remains will ultimately be deposited in a foreign land. I may lie on my death bed without a friend or relative to close my eyes but I shall have one satisfaction, at least, that my remembrance will not perish.

The death of Keats was widely reported, as was the epitaph he asked to have on his tombstone: 'Here lies one whose name was writ in water', less confident than Thackrah was he of the longevity of his fame. It seems likely that Thackrah was deeply affected by the loss of his contemporary from medical school, knowing as he did that his own health was likely to restrict the work he could do.

In the next few years – from 1824 to 1828 – he was also to suffer a number of personal tragedies. Fathering an illegitimate child lowered him in the esteem of some of his colleagues, and when he married in 1824 and had a daughter, his happiness was short-lived. His wife died within four years and his child died just a few months later. In addition, he was to lose his mother. But in this same period, he was also to pursue his ambition to teach, and he took on a number of apprentices. He gave popular lectures on physiology, and in 1826 he set up a private School of Anatomy in his own home; research has uncovered evidence that Thackrah's students turned resurrection men in order to provide themselves with the necessary subjects for dissection.

It was by establishing himself as the head of his own school, however, that he came into conflict with the surgeons at the infirmary. The senior medical men at the hospital were criticised as incompetent by the junior members, who were mainly apothecaries and mainly allied to Thackrah. Thackrah and Samuel Smith MRCS conducted an acrimonious debate in the pages of the Leeds newspapers, in which Thackrah, defending one of his pupils, wrote of the senior members: 'They have rendered themselves despicable in society for a talemaker is the skunk of every company he enters…. It would be easy to make them "the sewer of their own mess".'

In return, Samuel Smith, by all accounts a fine and well-respected surgeon, suggested that Thackrah would be wonderful as an actor in 'the inimitable Sheridan's play', and that his replies were little more than puffing up his own achievements at the expense of others more experienced and better trained than himself.

It is known that the two men were eventually reconciled, as essentially they agreed on the problems of child labour that existed in Leeds, but the spat highlights the high opinion Thackrah had of his own worth as a doctor, and as a teacher, and his following grew amongst the surgeons he trained. He was determined to make his name, and he continued to teach, and to research, despite his continuing poor health.

In 1830 he married again, to Grace Greenwood, and enjoyed calmer relationships with colleagues at the infirmary, this was a period within which he could find time to relax and rest.

This period was one in which the establishment of new schools of medicine was flourishing and in 1831 six surgeons and physicians of the infirmary and the dispensary, including Thackrah's antagonist, Samuel Smith, determined to establish a school in Leeds. Thackrah, as an exponent of systematic teaching based on his own training, was invited to co-operate and he agreed to merge his School of Anatomy with the new Leeds Medical School. He gave one of the lectures scheduled for the very first session on Tuesday 25 October 1831, and thereafter taught anatomy, physiology, pathology, and surgery.

Thackrah's work brought him into direct contact with medical problems directly attributable to the working conditions of the different trades in Leeds, particularly the many textile mills in the area, and remarkable, for a man in such poor health, in the year the Leeds Medical School was founded, he also published the first edition of his book on industrial diseases, which was to be extended and republished in 1832 as *The Effects of Arts, Trades and Professions and of civic states and habits of living on Health and Longevity with suggestions for removal of many of the agents which produce disease and shorten the duration of life*. In it he points out that the great wonders of the age, in both science and art, have an effect on the wider population, in both a physical and moral sense:

> *I refer to the health of fifty thousand persons, who spend their lives in the manufactories of Leeds and its neighbourhood or in allied and dependent occupations. I ask if these fifty thousand persons enjoy that vigour of body, which is ever a direct good and without which all other advantages are comparatively worthless?*

He insisted that an examination of the working conditions of these thousands of people was long overdue and that he hoped his work would raise awareness in the public mind.

He certainly achieved his aim; the book was a huge success, both in the United Kingdom and in America. A review in The Lancet stated:

> *In conclusion, we confidently recommend Mr Thackrah's work to the attention of the profession, among which we trust he will find some successful followers in the benevolent cause he thus invites others to pursue.*

The book made reference to more than one hundred trades common in Leeds at the time, including the problems experienced by child mill workers, deformed by the tasks they were required to perform, and miners affected by dust. Importantly, he made recommendations for change, directly contributing to the passing of the Factory Act in 1833, prohibiting the employment of children under 9 in the textile mills. Occupational Medicine as a discipline was established as a result.

Sadly, Thackrah was never able to follow his own best principles when it came to his own health. His relentless workload and desire to constantly revise and update his work, meant he ignored his failing condition and he died of tuberculosis on 23 May 1833, aged 38.

His work on preventative medicine was compared by some in importance to the work of his fellow surgeon–apothecary Edward Jenner on smallpox, and although his name is not so widely known now, his fame was secured, certainly in Yorkshire. An obituary appeared in the *Leeds Mercury*, summing up the nature of his character and achievements:

> *Distinguished by an ardent zeal in his profession, to which he devoted his mind with unremitting assiduity, and gifted with a sound judgement to weigh accurately the results of laborious and patient investigation, Mr Thackrah early rose to eminence…He will long be deeply lamented by the numerous individuals, who from experience if his talents were best able to appreciate them.*

Chapter 9

The Weekes letters – a country practice, a medical dynasty

he Weekes family letters, numbering 121 manuscript letters
exchanged between 1796 and 1803, offer a wonderful picture of the
life of a country doctor and his family in the late eighteenth and
early nineteenth centuries. From the medical matters discussed, it is clear
that the role of the country practitioner was one of a general practitioner.
Thomas Laffan quoted in *A Medical Student at St Thomas's Hospital 1801–
1802 The Weekes Family Letters* by John M.T. Ford states:

> *In the pure country, they* [surgeon-apothecaries] *are almost as
> exclusive attendants upon everyone, rich and poor. The lord who calls
> in the great gun, whether medical or surgical is, while in the country,
> almost entirely in the hands of general practitioners…but a time comes
> when difficulties far greater that those which either Dublin or London
> folk have to contend with assail patients, then the greatest lord no less
> than his meanest tenant is completely at the mercy of the skill and ability
> of the smallest village practitioner…*

Although written later in the nineteenth century, this was true of the lives
led in the village of Hurstpierpoint, near Brighton in Sussex at the turn of
the century.

The focus of the correspondence in the Weekes letters is Hampton
Weekes, elder son of Richard Weekes, surgeon-apothecary of Hurstpierpoint
and father and son write to each other frequently. There are also many letters
between Hampton Weekes and Owen Evans, a friend and medical student at
St Bartholomew's Hospital in London. The letters are a very rare resource,
as John M.T. Ford points out; very few letters from doctors have survived
in numbers. Other information can be found in account books, day books,
prescriptions and in shorter runs of letters, but these first-hand accounts of
the day-to-day life of both a student of medicine and his father's practice
are unique.

Hampton Weekes was the eldest child of Richard Weekes and his first wife, Charity, née Hampton. He was a pupil at the Merchant Taylors School between 1791 and 1796 and then returned to start his medical training, as surgeon-apothecary, presumably (and in the absence of any formal record) as an apprentice to his father. Between 1801 and 1803 when the most interesting letters are written, Hampton Weekes was in London working as an apothecary's pupil to Richard Whitfield of St Thomas's Hospital. In 1802 he became a member of the Royal College of Surgeons although he may not have intended to follow his father into practice at Hurstpierpoint; his letters refer to the possibility of joining the army or establishing himself in a different location and Ford has identified a Weekes in Brighton in 1805 and in Aberdeen in 1808, by which time Hampton had married Sarah Borrer, his childhood sweetheart. By 1810 he and his young family (his first son was born in 1808) were back in Hurstpierpoint, where he took on his father's work and fathered seven additional children, three of whom died in young adulthood. Two of his sons, however, followed him into the medical profession: Richard, qualifying in 1830, and George in 1838, becoming Surgeon to the Royal Sussex Militia Academy.

Hampton Weekes's brother, Richard (usually referred to as Dick), studied medicine and returned to work with Richard Snr before following Hampton as assistant to Whitfield at St Thomas's. He too is one of the key correspondents.

Life in a country practice

Richard Weekes Snr was a dedicated physician, regularly called in to give a second opinion where required, for which he charged one guinea. He attended the local large houses of the gentry, initially to treat the staff, but increasingly he was called upon to treat guests. John Ford maintains that the Weekes family are a good example of the evolution of the medical dynasty. Mrs Weekes in her role as wife to the local surgeon-apothecary was as important as the medical man himself. She would have maintained the house, administered the practice, looked after any apprentices and ensured that the doctors were fed at all hours. Sons were as important to the medical family as to the royals, and a good doctor's wife would 'bring them up in a way that would make them want to carry on the business rather than put them off medicine for life' (Ford p9).

The information held in the letters themselves is limited only as far as the correspondents were likely to take the most mundane, routine tasks for granted and leave a lengthy description of them out. Surgical cases, for example, were rather more likely to be 'exciting' or interesting enough to write about. It is indicative of the difference a medical man could make in medical cases, often the only treatment was supportive, and the mere presence of the doctor was reassuring, despite the few treatments that could make a genuine difference. We know he would have changed dressings and treated the minor cases – perhaps the digestive problems of those wealthy enough to over-indulge – on a regular basis without note.

Of the more serious medical cases, smallpox is most regularly mentioned and the vaccination regime suggested by Jenner (although still seeing much opposition from envious contemporaries) was used widely by doctors in the Sussex area. There is an enthusiasm for hearing all the latest on the subject from the London hospitals, and Hampton Weekes is keen to pass on advice to practitioners from Jenner himself, such as this relating to the speed with which the infected material used in vaccination is extracted:

> *Our Cowpock paper was finished being discussed, on Saturday eveng.*
> *last, it afforded me great entertainment as it would every practitioner,*
> *… Dr J. concludes from all he has been able to inform himself that if*
> *matter is not taken early either from ye Cow or any human subject that*
> *it is more probable you will have ye spurious pustule produced, that is*
> *after ye. 7th. or 8th. Day of Inocn … the matter containd in ye pustule*
> *undergoes a considerable change that is in a manner decomposed…*

Other medical conditions mentioned in brief include scarlatina (of which a number of children died), diphtheria, typhus, rheumatism (from which Richard Weekes Snr suffered), croup and tuberculosis, of the lungs, and of the knee.

Richard Snr was as dedicated to his poor patients as he was to the rich, and rode many miles in all weathers when necessary. His letters express his frustration at his own injury or illness that might take him from his patients. His was a business after all, and patients would soon look elsewhere for help.

With little impact to be made in the field of medicine (although some cases would become chronic, and therefore – with the necessity for continuing prescriptions – more lucrative) proficiency in surgery was, therefore, vital, and Ford notes how keen Richard Snr was to ensure Hampton attended to his surgical lectures and practice. Many of the emergency cases noted in the letters involve trauma of some kind. Accidental gunshot wounds shattering hands and blasting the abdomen required a rapid response. A child was badly burned after her clothes caught fire, requiring regular visits, and in a grim accident in July 1802, Dick Weekes wrote to his brother of his father's urgent ride out:

> ...*to Albourne to see one of ... Maskall's Children the Child fell into the petit* [lavatory or water closet] *and was Smothered and had been dead ¾ of an hour before my G=father arrived, the Stomach was distended with it, and he squeezed a good deal out of Mouth and Nose tried warm bath & cc all of no kind of use.*

This was so desperate a tragedy that it was reported in the local press (*Weekly Advertiser and Lewes Journal*, 2 August 1802) as 'On Sunday, a child, about two years old, was suffocated in the soil of a privy, into which it has accidentally fallen, at Albourne, near Hurstpierpoint [sic]'. In this period there were, sadly, so many ways to lose one's life.

Broken bones, concussions and sprains were regular occurrences in a country practice, and the sprained ankle suffered by Richard Weekes was particularly noteworthy, preventing him, as it did, from attending to his patients.

Other surgery seems quite remarkable at a time when so little was known of the complexities of the human body, and when no anaesthesia was available to prevent the agonies a patient must suffer. Richard Weekes wrote to Hampton on 18 November 1801 and recounted: 'I was sent for yesterday to the Pockneys at Cuckfield to make a new Anus in a girl about 14 months old the one she had was too near the Vagina & very small I made one accordingly...'

And on 27 November 1802, Dick Weekes wrote:

> ...*My father...is gone to Henfield to see a Girl who had an abscess opened a few Days ago under the Musc. Cutaneus Fems: on the upper side of the Thigh. It is not a Lumbar Abscess I believe. 1 Quart curdled Pus evacuated from the incision...*

Earlier that year, Dick had described an operation that for him was fraught with one difficulty, but which for the patient must have been unutterably painful:

> ...*the Bistory (surgical tool) you bought for me the other day & with which I operated on Mr Hodson for Fistula in Ano (a small tunnel that can develop near the anus and here 'where the opening into the Rectum was*

about 2 Inches up the Sinus') broke just as I was about half finish'd the operation just like a piece of glass I was for the moment much embarrass'd but taking out my Forceps & having a piece of Twine at hand I tied the piece of Bistory tight within the blades of the forceps & finish'd diving the Sphincter Ani Muscle. I did not press the point of it harder against my finger than was necessary to keep it steady, but it was too highly temperd & I think rather too slight, It shd. Bend rather than break, I will send it up to you to be renewed Gratis I hope, What an unpleasant circumstance – The Wound now Contracts the discharge is abated and it will soon be well…

Clearly, a surgeon was required to think on his feet when there was little but opiates and alcohol to keep the patient quiet.

The Weekes letters also offer an intimate look at the process of childbirth, which was a regular occurrence in the lives of a country parish, but one that was often complicated, dangerous, and fraught with tragic possibilities. The very poor usually managed a home delivery with no medical attendant present. In special cases where the family could afford to pay for a 'man-midwife' (which was frequently appended to the title 'surgeon-apothecary') the doctor was present, often for hours on end and with relatively poor financial reward. As previously noted; the Weekes family charged 15s for delivering a parish baby, but five guineas to a wealthier patient. However, for that sum the doctor would also have to attend daily (and in the example given the distance to cover was three miles) and if there were any 'false alarms' before the child was actually delivered there was no possibility of additional payment. The birth of a child, however, was often the start of a lifetime connection between the doctor and an entire family so the additional care was an investment in future business.

It was a challenging period in the life of doctor and patient, and at times Richard Weekes was present at five or six labours in a week. The lack of knowledge of antisepsis also made the women more vulnerable to puerperal, or 'childbed', fever an infection of the womb or other reproductive organs most often caused by delivery in unhygienic conditions. The onset of the fever usually started within the ten days after birth and after the infection took hold the woman could suffer an abscess, or localised infection from which she might recover, a spread of the infection to the veins in the pelvis, causing septicaemia and usually death, or peritonitis, as the infection spread through the abdomen up the fallopian tubes, causing a desperately painful death.

In Chapter 7 the work of Robert Storrs in the field of obstetrics highlights how little doctors knew of the causes of this frequently fatal infection. Indeed one letter from Richard to Hampton suggests that it was not always easy for a doctor of the period to establish whether childbirth was the cause of the fever at all, as a diagnosis of scarlet fever had been initially made in one case. Healthy women died quite unnecessarily, simply because the doctor did not know to scrub up thoroughly before delivery, or even use clean surgical tools. Many fevers were medically untreatable at that time, however, and it was not until the advent of antibiotics that fever, once contracted, could be effectively cured. The methods Richard Weekes used to treat women, apparently healthy before going into labour, are benign but useless:

> *Your next question is in respect of puerperal fever, here I have my doubts again I have seen many cases of great disorder in the System after Parturision (birth) as I suppose during the eight & twenty years that I have been in business I have been with between 2 & 3 thousand women in Labour, in some cases I have thought the lancet has been necessary in others gentle laxatives to clear the stomach and intestines, in others strong doses of chamomile tea drank often whereby perspiration has been excited particularly where there has been suppression of the lochia, with fomentatives* [such as a poultice], *Opiates & c ...these things at times apparently has been service ... at other times nothing has done any good whatever. I lost two young women of puerperal fever last year they had both very easy and natural labours. & where in good health before delivery but the weather was exceeding hot & in consequence everything about the women more inclined to be putrid and offensive...*

Rates of puerperal fever increased as the number of births were attended by medical men, and in hospital surroundings, where women gave birth close to one another and a doctor might move from one to another without washing his hands. In the late eighteenth and early nineteenth centuries, the number of women dying in childbirth ranged from fifty to one hundred per thousand births. In the twenty-first century, a woman is unlikely to die from a puerperal infection, principally due to the much-improved hygiene methods and the advent of the antibiotic.

Life as a medical student

Hampton Weekes was learning the art of medicine before the Apothecaries Act of 1815 came into being, and was therefore not obliged to attend a course of hospital lectures or spend time on the wards. However, the family recognised that in order to be a successful local general practitioner at this time, an education at a top hospital was a distinct advantage, socially as well as professionally. Here connections could be made, and an education by the top surgeons of the day, who in the first years of the nineteenth century were granted some celebrity status, would offer financial advantage later when introductions to local gentry were sought.

For Hampton, Richard Weekes was keen to provide as effective a medical education as possible, and would also require his son to support the medical education of his younger brother Dick, and the curiosity of his father, who wanted to be updated on all the latest medical techniques and provided with the newest equipment for his practice in Sussex. John M.T. Ford states: 'It would be hard to devise a better medical education than Hampton's', and so it seems useful to describe it here.

What was better, at that time, than to be born into a medical family? The career and the pressures of making a medical living were well known and the support structure already in place. Hampton was sent as a boarder to a good grammar school, returning to take up an apprenticeship with his father, who was by all accounts a competent and hardworking doctor and could offer his son proper practical experience (many of those who took on apprentices in this period were both incompetent and more likely to have their apprentices holding their horse outside the patient's home than invite them in to see medicine at work). He was then given the opportunity to train as an apprentice to apothecary Richard Whitfield at St Thomas's Hospital in London, which, when it combined with neighbouring Guy's Hospital in 1802 (to become the United Borough Hospitals), offered the best all-round medical education in the city.

At St Thomas's Hampton would have helped in the hospital's apothecary shop, where he would learn his Materia Medica. He would have had the first-hand experience of the dissecting rooms (see Chapter 3) and was undoubtedly familiar with the work of the resurrection men, or body snatchers. One of whom, named 'Jemmy', is mentioned in a letter home to his brother, and dated December 1801. In it he says:

> *I have one bit of news to tell my father, wh. Is that old Jemmy, one of ye. resurrection Men in his time was shot not more than 5 or 6 years ago, as he was at his usual employ in Deptford. He was shot by one of the Greenwich pensioners by a ball passing thro: his Head & He fell into the Coffin…*

It is particularly interesting that these men are spoken about almost with affection and certainly as a normal part of everyday life in the hospitals for generations.

He attended lectures in the theory of medicine and was lucky enough to live and work with the apothecary, who would be sure to keep him working in his free time.

The life of a medical student has been described in relation to their response to the dissecting room, and the many rumours that circulated regarding the behaviour of medical students in general. John M.T. Ford quotes an anonymous medical student as saying, '...there is a great deal too much gaming going forward. Billiards and cards consume most of the time of certain gentlemen'.

However, Ford is keen to point out that the letters sent home by Hampton Weekes, although undoubtedly censored for family consumption, do not indicate that his focus was on much other than his studies. Ford's work uncovered visits to Covent Garden and Drury Lane, parties and dances and nights sleeping on the floor of a willing friend. There is also evidence that he was fond of female company, but his childhood sweetheart, Sarah, was always at the forefront of his mind. Ford discovered that:

> his most risqué story is of the dog that got loose in the dissecting room ("...a nasty little dog was in the dissecting room shut up there for some experiment or other & made free with the Os Cuboides & the falanges of the little Toe, for wh. I have substituted part of another foot"), and his most shocking act was to prepare a penis to send home. ("I was ye. Other day favord with a Poenis from one of ye. Pupils, (pretty large)").

His background was to his advantage, however. With a father in regular correspondence, expecting much in return for his investment, and a brother keen to follow in his footsteps, he was unlikely to waver from the path set out for him.

The medical education Hampton Weekes received would not have been cheap. Sadly, there is no full account of the costs incurred by Hampton, or the family back in Hurstpierpoint. An early letter of September 1801 lists some of his expenses, including £12 12s for the lectures of William Babington, James Curry and an unknown Mr Roberts, and £9 9s for the lectures of Henry Cline. He purchased a desk for £1 10s and spent 14s on a gown and 13s on a 'case of scalpels'. Sundry expenses include a shilling for 'Adcock's maid', 5s on a 'jaunt to Deptford' and 2s on a 'pipe & a glass of Grog' with Charles Fixott, a fellow pupil of Whitfield.

As a comparison, the medical education necessary to ensure John Keats became qualified as an apothecary and able to start his education as a surgeon, is estimated to amount to a figure between £700 to £1,000, according to the recollection of his guardian Richard Abbey (who one would expect to have kept a clear account) or of Charles Brown, Keats's close friend. Current currency values would put the figure at around £50,000. However, Keats did not come from a medical family and would have had to pay £200 for an apprenticeship that was free to Hampton, and also pay for board and lodgings in London. He would also have had to buy books, which Hampton would have had access to in his father's library.

Ford does compare Weekes to other medical students over the period, and expenditure varies from £150 per annum in the Edinburgh of 1775, to £130 for just the winter session of 1828-29. Ford estimates that one year of residence and tuition at the United Hospitals of Guy's and St Thomas's in 1801 would have cost the Weekes family between £150 and £175, or about £8,000 today.

The Weekes family letters are full of interesting information about the life of a country practice, but their detail does not extend far into the medical cases Hampton Weekes would have been involved with during his training in London. Ford points out that when cases are mentioned, they are almost invariably surgical interventions, with a particular emphasis on those of Astley Cooper, whom Hampton Weekes admired, especially where the procedure involved the repair of a hernia. Surgical cases that interested him are often described in graphic detail, particularly when the reader remembers that the operations, usually only undertaken if they could be completed quickly, took place without any effective form of anaesthesia and the patient, therefore, remained conscious throughout:

> There is a case of Hydrocele [a collection of fluid in the scrotum] in Guys Hl. Wh. was operated on Monday last but there is a great degree of inflamm. Come on ye Scrotum is very much enlarged & inflamed looks very bad. They keep him in bed & lay ye. Scrotum on a little pillow... The same day... Cooper operated for Poplitaeal aneurism [an aneurysm behind the knee in a branch of the femoral artery] & ye. lower ligature 1st came off & afterward ye. upper one twice & ye. poor fellow had nearly blood to death Cooper was somewhat intimidated, ye. operation was 1 hour about, But ye man is tolerable. Adieu.

Interesting medical cases are occasionally mentioned, but they are very much 'out of the ordinary'. One particularly sad case (although Hampton refers the patient as 'a great imposter') is a middle-aged woman who regularly caused her lower arm to swell by tightening her necklace around the upper part:

> *her arm all below has been much inflamed and swelled to ye size of two Arms'. This was clearly a woman crying out for a very different kind of help, so determined was she that she 'caused great disorder in her constitution {…} produced simptomatic fever & very great irritation, Blisters, Leaches, Poulticing, with puncturing, &c has been had recourse to.*

Hampton judges her to be simply a woman keen to 'impose on ye. Charity' as it transpired that 'She has been doing the same in almost all ye. Hospitals about.'

Another case also indicates the practical way in which Hampton Weekes viewed a body and was keen to take any part of it that caught his fancy:

> *I was in the dead house inspecting two bodies the other day with Mr Davey; one was a cancerous affection (I stole his bladder), The other Man died on account of excessive delirium brought on from a great quantity of Gin being taken into the Stomach…He had not been in the hospital more than 4 days; the whole of wh. Time he was so violent as to be confined by straps & a straight jackett…*

It would be wonderful to have had had similar detail on the more routine cases that a medical student might come across and the cases for which medicines only were supplied, but the letters do offer one of the clearest pictures of the day-to-day life of a medical family; at home, at work and in training, and for that we must be grateful to John Ford for his hard work in researching them.

Conclusion

GPs are primary care doctors providing the first point of contact with the NHS for most people in their communities. GPs help patients by trying to identify problems they may have at an early stage which could be as varied as an infectious disease, cancer or a safeguarding issue. They are the trusted adults to whom patients first turn for advice and support. GPs also try wherever possible to maintain the health of patients through preventive care and health promotion...GPs treat conditions such as: hypertension, cardiovascular diseases, diabetes, asthma, arthritis, kidney disease and other chronic and long-term conditions emotional, stress-related and other mild to moderate psychiatric illnesses...

(NHS Health Careers)

The general practitioners of twenty-first-century Great Britain are put through a rigorous training programme that lasts years following an initial medical degree. We take them very much for granted. Whilst at the same time suggesting that we can rarely get an appointment when we want one, and that they cannot spend long enough with us when we do succeed in getting past the receptionist, that a home visit is out of the question. Research for this book has shown that those men of the late eighteenth century and early nineteenth century had to deal with the same problems. It was a profession that required dedication, commitment and hard work.

The many satirical cartoons of the era that depict the physicians as little more than quacks, bleeding their patients dry – almost literally as well as metaphorically – disguise the natures of many of the men who spent hours on the road treating their communities for little financial reward. They could not often compensate with that warm glow of success that results from aiding a complete recovery from serious illness; the available drugs were at best little more than comforting placebos, and many were essentially poisons, administered in ignorance of the effects of long-term usage. Life in many communities was short and brutal, and childhood diseases easily managed today regularly proved fatal. Yet these were men whose very presence could provide the comfort a patient needed.

Many of the surgeon–apothecaries were fascinated by the cause and spread of disease, and undertook their own research, often with few facilities and in the very little spare time they had. Men included in this book – such as Thomas Paytherus – undertook work that supported better-known names (in Paytherus's case this was Edward Jenner in the field of smallpox vaccination) and others, like Richard Storrs, noted practices that could improve the outcomes for many of his patients. Their contributions to the profession may not be well known, but they should not be dismissed.

Appendix 1

Treatments available to the surgeon-apothecary

There were a number of treatment options open to the surgeon-apothecary of the eighteenth and nineteenth centuries, many of them based on medicines and lotions made for centuries from plant sources. Many people were, unwittingly, taking sufficient doses of substances like mercury, and the opiate in laudanum, to permanently damage their health, cause addiction or, in the worst cases, death. The apothecary had to be careful of the quantities prescribed and mixed.

For those unable, or unwilling, to seek the help of a professional medical man in this period, there was always Dr William Buchan's *Domestic Medicine* to turn to, and no self-respecting household would be without at least some knowledge of the self-care they could undertake to avoid the most common, less serious, medical complaints.

This list includes common remedies used in general practice as well as some of Buchan's remedies (in italics), along with some home preparations of the time. Some of these substances still form the basis of over the counter treatments available to self-medicate in the twenty-first century.

Antimony – a metal, often used as an emetic (to make the patient sick).

Balsam – a medicinal tincture or drink.

Anodyne Balsam – used to ease pain, particularly of 'strains and rheumatic complaints'.

Take of white Spanish soap, one ounce; opium, unprepared, two drachms; rectified spirit of wine, nine ounces. Digest them together in a gentle heat for three days; then strain off the liquor, and add to it three drachms of camphor. (William Buchan Domestic Medicine 2nd edition 1785.)

Belladonna – a poisonous plant used as a gastrointestinal antispasmodic.

Bolus – a medicine rolled into bean-sized pill to be swallowed whole.

Bolus of Rhubarb and Mercury. Take of the best rhubarb, in powder, from a scruple to half a drachm; of calomel, from four to six grains; simple syrup, a sufficient quantity to make a bolus. This is a proper purge in hypochondriac constitutions; but its principal intention is to expel worms. Where a stronger purge is necessary, jalap may be used instead of the rhubarb.

Calomel – a white, tasteless powder containing mercury used as a purgative (or strong laxative).

Cataplasm – a poultice, and better known as a plaster spread over the skin for medical treatment.

Cathartics – a laxative or purgative.

Clyster – an enema.

Take jelly of starch, four ounces; linseed oil, half an ounce. Liquify the jelly over a gentle fire, and then mix in the oil. In the dysentery or bloody flux, this clyster may be administered after every loose stool, to heal the ulcerated intestines and blunt the sharpness of corroding humours. Forty or fifty drops of laudanum may be occasionally added; in which case, it will generally supply the place of the Astringent Clyster.

Collyrium – an eye lotion or powder.

Cupping (dry) – drawing of blood to the surface of the skin by means of a vacuum cup.

Cupping (wet) – removal of blood by vacuum cup after scoring the skin.

Decoction – medicine prepared by boiling ingredients, cooling and straining before allowing to clear.

Diaphoretic – a drug inducing perspiration.

Digitalis – extract of foxglove strengthening heartbeat with and reducing oedema.

Draught – a dose of liquid medicine.

Diuretic Draught. Take of the diuretic salt two scruples; syrup of poppies, two drachms; simple cinnamon-water and common-water, of each an ounce. This draught is of service in an obstruction or deficiency of urine.

Electuary – a sweetened pill.

Electuary for the Gonorrhoea. Take of lenitive electuary, three ounces; jalap and rhubarb, in powder, of each two drachms; nitre, half an ounce; simple syrup, enough to make an electuary. During the inflammation and tension of the urinary passages, which accompany a virulent gonorrhoea, this cooling laxative may be used with advantage. The dose is a drachm, or about the bulk of a nutmeg two or three times a-day; more or less, as may be necessary to keep the body gently open. An electuary made of cream of tartar and simple syrup will occasionally supply the place of this.

After the inflammation is gone off, the following electuary may used: Take of lenitive electuary, two ounces; balsam of capivi, one ounce; gum guaiacum and rhubarb, in powder, of each two drachms; simple syrup, enough to make an electuary. The dose is the same as of the preceding.

Elixir – where a tincture has one ingredient, an elixir has more than one.

Paregoric Elixir. Take of flowers of benzoin, half an ounce; opium, two drachms. Infuse in one pound of the volatile aromatic spirit, for four or five days, frequently shaking the bottle; afterwards strain the elixir. This is an agreeable and safe way of administering opium. It eases pain, allays tickling coughs, relieves difficult breathing, and is useful in many disorders of children, particularly the hooping cough. The dose to an adult is from fifty to a hundred drops.

Emetic – an agent inducing vomiting.

Emulsion – minute droplets of one liquid in another in which it is not soluble or able to be homogenised (such as oil and water).

Camphorated Emulsion. Take of Camphor, half a drachm; sweet almonds, half a dozen; white sugar, half an ounce; mint water, eight ounces. Grind the camphor and almonds well together in a stone mortar, and add by degrees the mint water; then strain the liquor, and dissolve in it the sugar.

In fevers, and other disorders which require the use of camphor, a table-spoonful of this emulsion may be taken every two or three hours.

Expectorant – increases ability to cough up bronchial mucous.

Fomentation – the application of hot moist substances to the body to ease pain.

Aromatic Fomentation – Take of Jamaica pepper, half an ounce; red wine, a pint. Boil them for a little, and then strain the liquor. This is intended, not only as a topical application for external complaints, but also for relieving the internal parts. Pains of the bowels, which accompany dysenteries and diarrhoeas, flatulent colics, uneasiness of the stomach, and reachings to vomit, are frequently abated by fomenting the abdomen and region of the stomach with the warm liquor.

Gr – a grain (a measure of weight). There are around 440 grs to one ounce.

Gtt – a drop (measurement).

Humoral imbalance – the ascribing of illness, and disease, to an abnormal condition of the humours (fluids) in the body.

Infusion – a medicine made by pouring boiling water onto ingredients such as plants.

Infusion for The Palsy. Take of horse-radish root shaved, mustard seed bruised, each four ounces; outer rind of orange-peel, one ounce. Infuse them in two quarts of boiling water, in a close vessel, for twenty-four hours. In paralytic complaints, a tea-cupful of this warm stimulating medicine may be taken three or four times a-day. It excites the action of the solids, proves diuretic, and, if the patient be kept warm, promotes perspiration.

Julep – a draught with a syrup added. Most usually called 'mixtures' in the nineteenth century.

Musk Julep. Rub half a drachm of musk well together with half an ounce of sugar, and add to it, gradually, of simple cinnamon and pepper-mint water, each two ounces; of the volatile aromatic spirit, two drachms. In the low state of nervous fevers, hiccuping, convulsions, and other spasmodic affections; two table-spoonfuls of this julep may be taken every two or three hours.

Laudanum – tincture of opium.

Mixture – water based medicine with two or more ingredients.

Astringent Mixture. Take simple cinnamon-water and common water, of each three ounces; spirituous cinnamon–water, an ounce and a half; Japonic confection, half an ounce. Mix them. In dysenteries which are not of long standing, after the necessary evacuations, a spoonful or two of this mixture may be taken every four hours, interposing every second or third day a dose of rhubarb.

Ointment – can be stiff 'pastes' and more liquid 'creams'.

Eye Ointments. Take of hogs' lard prepared, four ounces; white wax, two drachms; tutty prepared, one ounce; melt the wax with the lard over a gentle fire, and then sprinkle in the tutty, continually stirring them till the ointment is cold.

Pill – small round solid medicine, originally used for medicines requiring only small doses.

Pills for the Jaundice. Take of Castile soap, succotorine aloes, and rhubarb, of each one drachm. Make them into pills with a sufficient quantity of syrup or mucilage.

These pills, as their title expresses, are chiefly intended for the jaundice, which, with the assistance of proper diet, they will often cure. Five or six of them may be taken twice a day, more or less, as is necessary to keep the body open. It will be proper, however, during their use, to interpose now and then a vomit of ipecacuanha or tartar emetic.

Powders – medicine taken in thin fluid or in a syrup.

Powder for The Tape-worm. – Early in the morning the patient is to take in any liquid, two or three drachms, according to his age and constitution, of the root of the male fern reduced into a fine powder. About two hours afterwards, he is to take of calomel and resin of scammony, each ten grains; gum gamboge, six grains. These ingredients must be finely powdered and given in a little syrup, honey, treacle, or any thing that is most agreeable to the patient. He is then to walk gently about, now and then drinking a dish of weak green tea, till the worm is passed. If the powder of the fern produces nausea, or sickness, it may be removed by sucking the juice of an orange or lemon.

Quinine – extract from bark of cinchona tree used to treat malaria.

Sal volatile – solution of ammonium carbonate in alcohol (smelling salts).

Scarification – scratching the skin with a number of blades.

Setons – threads inserted under the skin to cause a discharge of pus.

Sinapism – a mustard plaster or poultice to treat inflammation or reduce irritation.

Stupe – a piece of soft cloth or cotton wool dipped in hot water and used to make a poultice .

Tincture – solution or liquid in alcohol.

Compound Tincture of Senna – Take of senna, one ounce; jalap, coriander seeds, and cream of tartar, of each half an ounce. Infuse them in a pint and a half of French brandy for a week; then strain the tincture, and add to it four ounces of fine sugar. This is an agreeable purge, and answers all the purposes of the Elixir salutis, and of Daffy's Elixir. The dose is from one to two or three ounces

Tinct. Opii – opium in alcohol solution.

Trephine – a surgical instrument for boring hole in the skull.

Venesection – the removal of a volume of blood as a treatment for certain blood disorders by cutting a vein and catching the blood in a bowl.

Waters – the basis of many juleps, or mixtures. Similar to infusion.

Pennyroyal Water. Take of pennyroyal leaves, dried, a pound and a half; water, from a gallon and a half to two gallons. Draw off by distillation one gallon. This water possesses, in a considerable degree, the smell, taste, and virtues of the plant. It is given in mixtures and juleps to hysteric patients. An infusion of the herb in boiling water answers nearly the same purposes.

Appendix 2

Some common complaints

Abscess – pus in tissues or other body parts (often in the mouth) most often caused by bacteria. Symptoms included pain and inflammation. Other terms used include 'boil' or 'furuncle'.

Ague – malarial or other intermittent fever – with symptoms including fever and sweating. Characterised by remission and regular recurrence.

Anaemia – low number of red blood cells, frequently caused by a lack of iron. Not formally recognised until 1849, anaemia regularly afflicted those already subject to bleeding by doctors for other complaints.

Apoplexy – a stroke or cerebral haemorrhage, often causing paralysis.

Atrophy – this term refers to a wasting disease, not always identified, but which caused the body to degenerate, a symptom of any illness that lowered the appetite or prevented movement.

Biliousness – nausea, abdominal discomfort, headache, and constipation. A term still used, informally, to describe a condition attributed to the liver (from the 'bile' it produces).

Brain fever – would include meningitis and other illnesses diagnosed as an inflammation of the brain.

Bright's Disease – inflammation of the kidneys first described in 1827 by Richard Bright (1789–1858) working at Guy's hospital in London.

Bronchial asthma – a breathing disorder often caused by environmental factors (such as dust, or an allergic reaction to animals). Symptoms include acute spasms of the bronchial tubes, difficulty in breathing, wheezing and coughing. The causes were already recognised in this period, but there was little in the way of treatment and even today it can prove fatal.

Cancer – a malignant and invasive tumour. Physicians had recognised that cancerous tumours grew, sometimes rapidly until death became inevitable. Tumours that had ulcerated were also identified by early physicians and if caught early a surgical intervention could prove successful (as in the case of Fanny Burney, who described the mastectomy performed to treat her breast cancer in September 1811). However, Dr Johnson, in the mid-eighteenth century, in defining cancer as 'A virulent swelling or sore, not to be cured' was largely correct. It is a brave doctor, even now, who can claim to 'cure' cancer.

Cancrum Otis or Canker – an ulcer on the cheek and lip, most often found in children fed a poor diet. It could cause gangrene, putrid saliva and teeth would fall out. Sometimes appearing as a result of poor immunity following another acute illness, it could be fatal.

'Canine madness'– rabies or hydrophobia – caused by the bite of an infected dog. The symptoms included fever, hallucinations and a morbid fear of water. Death was inevitable and horrible to witness.

Catalepsy – a seizure or a trance-like state.

Catarrh – inflammation of the mucous membrane, most notably of head and throat causing a runny nose, watering eyes and cough. Catarrh could be attached to other illnesses, such as bronchitis (as in 'Bronchial catarrh') and croup (known as 'suffocative catarrh'. The appearance of catarrh in other parts of the body could be described as 'gleet' (in the urethra) or leukorrhea (from the vagina).

Child bed fever – also known as 'puerperal fever'. A type of septicaemia, which was a serious risk factor in childbirth before doctors recognised the importance of good hygiene during the birth of a baby.

Cholera – before the first outbreak of 'cholera morbus' in England in 1831, a milder 'gastroenteritis' was referred to as English cholera, and was usually less virulent. Cholera morbus (or simply, 'cholera') produced symptoms such as increasing and painful diarrhoea and vomiting accompanied by intense retching, causing unbearable pains. There would also be severe pain in the limbs, and the skin could turn a shade of blue or grey. Doctors were divided in their view of the cause of the disease and often had to watch their patients die within hours.

Chorea – also referred to as 'St Vitus' Dance' due to the involuntary, spasms often affecting the face, hands and feet.

Colic – a pain in the abdomen or bowels. It is still often seen in babies in the first three months of life and was unlikely to prove fatal. A 'renal colic' refers to a disease in the kidney, and 'biliary colic' to gallstones passing into the bile duct.

Congestion – when seen in a doctor's notes it refers to 'an accumulation of blood or other fluid in a body part or blood vessel' and is not a disease in itself, but a symptom.

Consumption – most frequently applied to pulmonary tuberculosis and could also be referred to as marasmus and phthisis. The term pulmonary tuberculosis was first used in the early twentieth century.

Convulsion – often used in the descriptions of epilepsy and caused by frequently violent, involuntary muscular contractions the body. Seizures can also be caused by conditions such as diabetes and in this period were often all referred to as 'falling sickness' or fits.

Corruption – another word for infection.

Costiveness – another word for constipation.

Croup – childhood condition affecting the windpipe (trachea), the airways to the lungs (the bronchi) and the voice box (larynx). It causes affected children to have a 'barking' cough and to make a harsh sound when they breathe in. It can block the airway and cause difficulty breathing.

Cystitis – inflammation of the bladder.

Debility – a description of a weakness or feebleness of the body.

Diarrhoea – the frequent passing of watery stools. It may be caused by a bowel infection and was a key symptom in diseases such as cholera.

Diphtheria – acute bacterial infection that mainly affecting the nose and throat, and highly contagious, being spread by coughs and sneezes, contact with someone with diphtheria or even with bedding or clothing. It was only called Diphtheria from 1826, but was known well before that as 'Boulogne sore throat' (amongst other names), as it was believed to come from the Continent.

Dropsy – oedema or quantities of fluid in tissue or body cavities. In the abdomen, it is referred to as ascites and can be a symptom of a number of illnesses. In the brain, it is referred to as hydrocephalus.

Dysentery – a highly infectious inflammation of the intestine. The symptoms are bloody diarrhoea, abdominal cramps and vomiting. It was a common problem for armies abroad.

Dyspepsia – acid indigestion or heartburn.

Enteric fever – a common term for typhoid fever.

Enteritis – inflammation of the bowel.

Epilepsy – seizures starting in the brain.

Erysipelas – an acute bacterial infection causing burning, dark red patches on the skin, and also known as St Anthony's fire, and commonly used as another term for cellulitis (which affects the deeper layers of skin).

Fistula in Ano – a small channel that can develop between the end of the bowel and the skin near the anus.

French Pox – a sexually transmitted disease and former name for syphilis.

Gangrene – loss of blood supply causes body tissue to die. It typically starts in the toes, feet, fingers and hands and can result in the loss of limbs, and ultimately death. Anyone suffering from this 'mortification' needed the amputation of the affected body part or its spread would be fatal.

Goitre – a swelling of the thyroid gland, appearing in the neck, caused by a shortage of iodine in the diet.

Gout – where small crystals form inside and around the joints, causing sudden attacks of severe pain and swelling. It is often found in the feet, causing severe discomfort. In the eighteenth and nineteenth centuries, it was often caused by drinking too much port or other fortified wine.

Gravel – small stones in the kidneys that pass along the ureter to the bladder. They are normally excreted in the urine, but when bigger can become stuck, causing excruciating pain.

Grippe – an eighteenth-century term for influenza, from the French 'La Grippe'.

Haemorrhoids – also known as 'piles' this was a common complaint causing swollen veins located around the anus or in the lower rectum.

Hives – itchy, red wheals on the skin, rarely fatal and often caused by an allergy.

Hysteritis – inflammation of the womb, causing severe pain deep in the pelvis.

Inanition – this word generally refers to weakness and exhaustion, caused by lack of food or any form of nourishment, i.e. starvation.

Infection – invasion of an organism's body tissues by disease-causing agents. The microorganisms multiply causing a reaction in the tissues and the production of toxins underpinning a disease. In this period (1750–1850) there was little understanding of the true cause of infectious disease, which was believed to be caused by 'effluvia' or 'miasma' (invisible, noxious vapours). Infections were often spread by doctors themselves, unaware of the principles of antisepsis.

Inflammation – a descriptive term for the protective response to injury or disease. Descriptions of diseases resulting in inflammation end with the term 'itis', such as 'appendicitis'.

Intussusception – the slipping of one part of the intestine into another. It causes cramping pain in the abdomen, nausea and vomiting.

Jail fever – another name for typhus.

Jaundice – causing the skin and eyes to turn yellow, faeces to become pale and urine dark, it is usually caused by liver disorders but some believed it could be brought on by the consumption of unripe fruit or the drinking of cold water.

Kidney stone – also referred to as 'Stone' and generally the larger and more obstructive cousin of 'gravel'. When the stone causes an obstruction it causes renal colic, with intense pains, urinary urgency, restlessness, haematuria (blood in the urine), sweating, nausea, and vomiting.

Leprosy – a long-lasting disease described by Dr Johnson as 'a loathsome distemper, which covers the body with a kind of white scales'.

Lockjaw – the popular term for tetanus, this is an infection causing acute muscle spasms, which start in the face and becoming widespread. It is caused by bacteria often found in soil and manure. It was not possible to vaccinate against tetanus until the 1920s.

Mania – another term for insanity.

Marasmus – severe undernourishment in children, causing very low weight, dry skin and poor muscle development.

Measles – highly infectious viral illness that can be very unpleasant and which can sometimes lead to serious complications. In the eighteenth and nineteenth centuries it was frequently fatal, especially in children.

Melancholia – the name comes from the Greek and literally means 'black bile', an imbalance of which was believed to cause symptoms that we would now associate with clinical depression.

Morbus – the Latin word for 'disease' and the means of identifying where the illness is sited. 'Morbus cordis' is heart disease, for example.

Nephritis – inflammation of the kidneys.

Palsy – referring to various types of paralysis, often accompanied by weakness and the loss of feeling and uncontrolled body movements such as shaking. Dr Johnson defined palsy as 'a privation of motion or feeling or both, proceeding from some cause below the cerebellum, joined with coldness, flaccidity, and at last wasting of the parts'. Palsy could refer to injury as well as illness in this period and the condition 'shaking palsy', later named after Dr James Parkinson who identified the condition (see Chapter 7).

Phrenitis – another term for an inflammation of the brain.

Pleurisy – inflammation of the 'pleura' lining the chest cavity. Symptoms include fever, dry cough and pain, and the possible production of fluid collecting in the pleural cavity.

Pneumonia – originating from the Greek, meaning 'lung', pneumonia had been identified for centuries before the bacteria causing it were identified in the late nineteenth century. Symptoms include a cough, fever, shortness of breath, stabbing chest pain on breathing, and in the elderly, confusion.

Puerperal fever – see also 'childbed fever', arising from childbirth. It is caused by bacterial infection and was frequently fatal until the advent of antibiotic treatment in the mid-twentieth century. Robert Storrs (see Chapter 7) was one of the first doctors to recognise his own role in the spread of the disease, carrying the infection from person to person on his body and clothing.

Pus – thick yellow or green liquid, made up of dead white blood cells, bacteria and tissue waste, produced in infected tissue.

Quinsy – acute inflammation of the tonsils that causes a pus-filled abscess between a tonsil and the throat wall. It was a serious illness that could cause death by suffocation.

Rheumatism – inflammation and pain in the joints and muscles, which was also known as 'Screws'.

Rickets – condition affecting bone development in children, which causes the bones to become soft and weak, causing deformities. It is usually caused by an extreme and prolonged vitamin D deficiency.

Rupture – A break or tear in any organ (such as the spleen) or soft tissue (such as the Achilles tendon).

Scarlatina, or Scarlet fever – a contagious disease of childhood caused by the Streptococcus bacterium, which can develop after a sore throat or a skin infection, such as impetigo, caused by streptococcus bacteria. Many serious cases resulted in death during this period, but antibiotics have made the disease much rarer.

Scrofula – cervical tuberculosis or swelling of the lymph nodes in the neck caused by tuberculosis, this was usually a disease of childhood or young adulthood. Also referred to as 'King's Evil', in the Middle Ages it was believed the touch from royalty could cure the condition.

Scurvy – a vitamin C deficiency common on long voyages and the scourge of early eighteenth century sailors. In 1753, British naval surgeon James Lind discovered that by simply eating citrus fruit, the condition could be avoided, although the British Navy did not adopt the regular practice until the 1790s. The symptoms of scurvy include a feeling of general ill-health, bleeding gums and haemorrhaging under the skin.

Smallpox – also known as variola. This was a highly contagious, disfiguring and frequently fatal disease with no cure, or successful treatment; Symptoms included fever, headache and severe fatigue, followed within days by flat, red spots, eventually covering the whole body. They filled with pus and scabbed over leaving deep scars. Edward Jenner developed a successful vaccine in the 1790s.

Stranguary – blockage or irritation at the base of the bladder, resulting in severe pain and a strong desire to urinate, which can be associated with kidney stones or prostate problems.

Suppuration – when used in medical records or books this refers to the production of pus, perhaps in a sore or wound.

Syphilis – a contagious sexually transmitted disease, which lasts many years and goes through three stages: primary, secondary and tertiary. It is only infectious in the primary stage, and can be passed to the foetus during pregnancy.

Tetanus – see 'Lockjaw'.

Thrush – disease causing whitish spots and ulcers on the membranes of the mouth, tongue, and throat caused by a parasitic fungus, Candida albicans. It was known to affect weak children and elderly people in poor health.

Typhoid fever – infectious, frequently fatal, disease causing fever and abdominal pain. Often contracted by eating contaminated food or drink, it also causes a skin rash develops and potential delirium. It should not be confused with Typhus (see below), which it resembles, and is also called enteric fever. Some people carry and pass on the disease without any symptoms themselves.

Typhus – Acute, infectious disease caused by several microorganisms, transmitted by lice and fleas. It causes a sudden, severe headache often followed by fever, a pink or red rash and vomiting. There is a pain in the abdomen, joints and muscles and a cough. It was also referred to as 'typhus fever', 'jail fever' and 'ship fever', largely because those in confined spaces were prone to contracting the disease from the body lice of those with whom they were incarcerated with.

Ulcer – an open sore, which can be found on an external (as on a leg) or internal (as in the mouth, or in the stomach) surface of the body. It is caused by a break in the skin or mucous membrane which fails to heal.

Undulant fever – or 'brucellosis', an infectious fever contracted from contaminated milk.

Venereal disease – now referred to as STIs or sexually transmitted diseases, these are infections commonly spread by vaginal intercourse, anal sex and oral sex. Syphilis and gonorrhoea were two of the most common venereal diseases in Europe, frequently believed to have been spread by sailors travelling the world. Syphilis was especially serious, as although it was only contagious in its 'primary stage', lasting just a few months, it could, in later stages, affect the brain and spinal cord, and could be passed to the unborn child.

In the eighteenth and nineteenth centuries, mercury, arsenic and sulphur were commonly used to treat venereal disease, which often resulted in serious side effects and many people died of mercury poisoning. The first known effective treatment for syphilis wasn't introduced until 1910.

Whooping Cough – also known as 'chincough'; a cough with a particular 'whooping' sound that became significant from the eighteenth century onwards. It was believed to be confined to children and could prove fatal, particularly in poorer parts of the country.

Appendix 3

Women in medicine

The medical profession has been dominated by men throughout history, even though women have always been relied upon to provide medical care. In the period 1750 to 1850, the teaching of medicine changed but certainly did not permit the training of women as doctors. A university education was required to practice as a physician and women were not accepted into universities, so that avenue was denied to them. Neither could they formally undertake the apprenticeships necessary to train as a surgeon–apothecary, or walk the wards of the schools attached to large teaching hospitals. Thus it was impossible to obtain the required licence to practice.

Women had always provided medical care, however, either in the home, as a village herbalist, or as a midwife for example. Paintings in tombs and temples of Ancient Egypt suggest Egyptian women undertook surgical procedures, particularly those needed by women, such as caesarean sections and even the removal of breast cancer. Historians of Rome mention women as physicians. In the Middle Ages, Nuns were active in providing medical care and were key to health care in the medieval period, when monks had been prohibited from bloodletting and undertaking certain surgical procedures. The Christian Abbess, author Hildegard of Bingen, established nursing orders and convent infirmaries and her practice allowed her to gain diagnostic skills, and the ability to combine a physical treatment with her 'spiritual healing' and holistic approach.

Women acted as sick-nurses, and wet nurses (breastfeeding another woman's baby) and, perhaps taught by an apothecary father or brother, could often undertake minor surgical procedures. The law permitted women to inherit their husband's apothecary business and many carried on with some success, the time spent helping in the apothecary's shop and the education required to mix the medicines deemed to be equivalent to an apprenticeship. According to Judith Woolf however, most women of this era did not keep a record of their lives – or at least few survive. It was only when she experienced some difficulty in her life that a woman's name will appear in official documents, so it difficult to gauge in what numbers these female apothecaries practised.

Midwives could not form themselves into a guild but were required to be licenced by the ecclesiastical authorities, and in London created a programme of training not unlike an apprenticeship. In Tudor and Stuart times it was seen as a philanthropic act to undertake medical work in the local community and many quite wealthy local women undertook the medical care for their communities. However, these women faced a lot of discrimination and criticism from the men in the medical profession, and at the height of the witch hunts, were at risk of malicious accusation and arrest.

As previously discussed, in the eighteenth century surgeon-apothecaries were becoming man-midwives and were gradually usurping women in this traditional role. It was a continued downgrading of a woman's role in the delivery of medical care.

In the eighteenth and nineteenth centuries, it was common for a man to write a manual debunking traditional and folk medicine as unscientific and based on myth. Science was seen as the way to good health and science was, then at least, a man's world.

There is a watercolour in the Wellcome Library with the title 'The village doctress distilling eyewater'. It shows a middle-aged female medical practitioner emptying her bladder into a funnel, over a distilling bottle. There is another, seemingly younger female assistant doing the same into a barrel, and a cat urinates on the ground. The sign in the window says 'Humours in the eyes effectually cured by Deborah Pisillan' and the implication is that she is using her own urine to make a medicine to be rubbed into the eyes to cure what might be cataracts. It is probably by the artist and caricaturist Thomas Rowlandson, well known for lampooning the medical profession of the period. The fact that his subject here is a grotesquely drawn woman, and with what we know now of the difficulties women faced in the profession, this cartoon seems somewhat less amusing than some of those he drew of overweight physicians living off the fat of their wealthy clients.

In the mid-nineteenth century, nurses such as Florence Nightingale and Mary Seacole commanded the respect of many medical practitioners, and nursing was promoted as a respectable profession for young women. However, society accepted nursing because it was seen as a professional extension of a woman's 'natural' caring and nurturing role. There was no such acceptance of women becoming doctors, and indeed even the breakthrough made by Nightingale, and the development of 'Nightingale Nurses' did not take place during the period covered by this book.

But for some women, a nursing role was not enough and they were determined to be part of the medical profession, even if they had to take extraordinary steps to do so. In order to practise as a doctor, Margaret Ann Bulkley (1795-1865) lived as a man, named James Barry, to train and practise as a military surgeon, a role she maintained for forty-six years. Her family were behind her, and her arrival at medical school, as a man, was orchestrated by her uncle to enable her to fulfil her ambition. James was exceptional, however, and worked for many years as a British Army surgeon, serving in India and Cape Town. Florence Nightingale once described this slight, apparently quite feminine doctor as 'the most hardened creature I ever met', and it was only when he died of dysentery in 1865 that the truth was revealed. The army was so embarrassed that Margaret was officially buried as a man.

By the middle of the century, Elizabeth Blackwell has qualified, albeit having studied in Geneva, and in 1873 Elizabeth Garrett Anderson gained membership of the British Medical Association. The fight was not over, though – in the United Kingdom Garrett Anderson remained the sole female doctor for a further nineteen years, whilst the BMA wrangled with the challenge of admitting more women into training.

Bibliography

Books

Bates, A.W., *The Anatomy of Robert Knox: Murder, Mad Science and Medical Regulation in Nineteenth-Century Edinburgh* (Sussex Academic Press, 2010)

Baxter, Eric, *Dr Jephson of Leamington Spa* (Warwickshire Local History Society, 1980)

Beardsley, Martyn & Bennett, Nicholas eds., *'Gratefull to Providence': The Diary and Accounts of Matthew Flinders, Surgeon, Apothecary and Man-Midwife, 1775-1802* (Boydell Press, 2007)

Brown, John W., *The Streatham Grave Robbers: A Tale of Attempted Body Snatching in Streatham in 1814* (Local History Publications, 1998)

Buchan, William, *Domestic Medicine: or, A treatise on the prevention and cure of diseases, by regimen and simple medicines: with an appendix, containing a dispensatory for the use of private practitioners* (Philadelphia, 1784)

Burch, Druin, *Digging up the Dead: The Life and Times of Astley Cooper, an Extraordinary Surgeon* (Chatto & Windus, 2007)

Bynum W. F., & Porter, Roy, *William Hunter and the Eighteenth-Century Medical World* (Cambridge University Press, 2002)

Cameron, Hector Charles, *Mr. Guy's Hospital, 1726-1948* (Longmans, Green, 1954)

Cody, Lisa Forman, *Birthing the Nation: Sex, Science, and the Conception of Eighteenth-Century Britain* (Oxford University Press, 2005)

De Almeida, Hermione, *Romantic Medicine and John Keats* (Oxford University Press 1990)

Digby, Anne, *Making a Medical Living: Doctors and Patients in the English Market for Medicine, 1720-1911* (Cambridge University Press, 2002)

Flude, Kevin, & Herbert, Paul, *The Apothecary, Herbs and the Herb Garret* (The Old Operating Theatre Museum & Herb Garret Exhibition Book, 2012)

Ford, John M. T., *A Medical Student at St. Thomas's Hospital, 1801-1802: Weekes, Hampton, 1780-1855* (Wellcome Institute for the History of Medicine, 1987)

Gittings, Robert, *John Keats* (Little, Brown, 1968)

Goellnicht, Donald C., *The Poet-Physician: Keats and Medical Science* (University of Pittsburgh Press, 1984)

Hazard S., *A candid inquiry into the education, qualifications and offices of a surgeon-apothecary* (James Lucas, 1800)

Lennox, Suzie, *Bodysnatchers: Digging Up the Untold Stories of Britain's Resurrection Men* (Pen and Sword, 2016)

Loudon, Irvine, *Medical Care and the General Practitioner 1750-1850* (Clarendon Press, 1986)

MacDonald, Helen, *Human Remains: Dissection and its Histories* (Yale University Press, 2006)

Meiklejohn, A., *The Life, Work and Times of Charles Turner Thackrah, Surgeon and Apothecary of Leeds (1795-1833)* (E. & S. Livingstone, 1957)

Mitchell, Piers ed., *Anatomical Dissection in Enlightenment England and Beyond : Autopsy, Pathology, and Display* (Ashgate, 2012)

Morgan, Anna, ''A beautiful, but seductive science' or 'strange and revolting work'?: Medical student's experiences of dissection between 1830 and 1880.' (Academic Dissertation, Wellcome Trust Centre for the History of Medicine at University College London, 2001)

Motion, Andrew, *Keats* (Faber & Faber, 1998)

Newman, Charles Edward Kingsley, *The Evolution of Medical Education in the Nineteenth Century* (Oxford University Press, 1957)

Parkinson, James, 'The Hospital Pupil; or, an Essay Intended to Facilitate the Study of Medicine & Surgery' 1800 (H.D. Symonds, 1800)

Parkinson, James, *The villager's friend and physician, or, A familiar address on the preservation of health, and the removal of disease, on its first appearance* (1804)

Pierpoint, William S. *Keats, Stephens and Mackereth: The Unparallel Lives of Three Medical Students* (The Stephens Collection, 2010)

Porter, Roy, *Blood & Guts: A Short History of Medicine* (Penguin Books, 2002)

Porter, Roy, *Health for Sale: Quackery in England, 1660-1850* (Manchester University Press, 1989)

Quigley, Christine, *Dissection on display: cadavers, anatomists, and public spectacle* (McFarland & Co., 2012)

Rance, Caroline, *The Quack Doctor: Historical Remedies for all your Ills* (The History Press, 2013)

Roe, Nicholas, *John Keats: A New Life* (Yale University Press, 2012)

Richardson, Ruth, *Death, Dissection and the Destitute* (Phoenix, 2001)

Swann, James Blake Bailey, *The Diary of a Resurrectionist, 1811-1812: to which are added an account of the resurrection men in London and a short history of the passing of the Anatomy Act* (Sonnenschein & Co., 1896)

Tooth, John S. H., *Humane and Heroic: the Life and Love of a 19th Century Country Doctor* (John S. H. Tooth, 2007)

Thomas, Amanda J, *Cholera: The Victorian Plague* (Pen and Sword Books, 2015)

Wise, Sarah, *The Italian Boy: Murder and Grave-Robbery in 1830s* (Random House, 2012)

Journals

Barnard, John, ''The Busy Time': Keats's Duties at Guy's Hospital from Autumn 1816 to March 1817', *Romanticism*, Vol. 13, No. 3 (2007), pp. 199-218

Connor H, & Clark D. M., 'Thomas Paytherus (1752-1828): Entrepreneurial surgeon-apothecary and ardent Jennerian', *Journal of Medical Biography*, 21 (3) (Aug 2013), pp. 169-79

Dunn, P. M., 'Dr William Buchan (1729–1805) and his Domestic medicine Archives of Disease in Childhood - Fetal and Neonatal Edition' (2000), pp. 71-73

Epstein,Joseph ,'The Medical Keats', *The Hudson Review*, Vol. 52, No. 1 (Spring, 1999), pp. 44-64

Hamilton, Bernice, 'The Medical Profession in the Eighteenth Century', *The Economic History Review*, New Series Vol. 4, No. 2 (1951), pp. 141-169

Knott, John, 'Popular Attitudes to Death and Dissection in Early Nineteenth Century Britain: The Anatomy Act and the Poor', *Labour History*, No. 49 (Nov 1985), pp. 1-18

Lewis, Patrick A, 'James Parkinson: The Man Behind the Shaking Palsy', *Journal of Parkinson's Disease*, 2 (2012), pp. 181–7

Rivlin, J.J., 'Getting a Medical Qualification in England In The Nineteenth Century', http://www.evolve360.co.uk/data/10/docs/09/09rivlin.pdf

Ross, Ian, & Urquhart Ross, Carol, 'Body Snatching in the Nineteenth Century Britain: From Exhumation to Murder', *British Journal of Law and Society*, Vol. 6, No.1 (Summer 1979), pp. 108-18

Tomkins, Alannah, 'Who were his peers? The social and professional milieu of the provincial surgeon-apothecary in the late-eighteenth century', *Journal of Social History*, Vol. 44, (3) (2011), pp. 915-35

White, R.S. "Like Esculapius of Old' Keats's Medical Training', *The Keats-Shelley Review*, Vol.12 (1998) - Issue 1

Websites

http://thequackdoctor.com/

http://britainsforgottenbodysnatchers.blogspot.co.uk

https://janeaustensworld.wordpress.com/tag/regency-medicine/

http://mikerendell.com/tag/matters-medical/

http://www.thornber.net/medicine/html/medgloss.html

http://www.rootsweb.ancestry.com/~memigrat/diseases.html

http://www.britishnewspaperarchive.co.uk/

http://wellcomelibrary.org/

http://www.oldbaileyonline.org/

http://munksroll.rcplondon.ac.uk/ (Lives of the fellows is part of the Royal College of Physicians website

http://www.apothecaries.org/

TheHunterianMuseumhttps://www.rcseng.ac.uk/museums-and-archives/hunterian-museum

The John Johnson Collection of Printed Ephemera http://www.bodleian.ox.ac.uk/johnson

Index